A BREAST CANCER MEMOIR
BY THEDRA CULLAR-LEDFORD

DRAWING THE EYE TO NOTHINGNESS

Design: Stephen Cullar-Ledford
ISBN: 978-0-692-41223-7
Drawing the Eye to Nothingness: A Breast Cancer Memoir

Originally published in 2015 by Independence Art Press, Houston, Texas

Printed and bound in the United States of America.

Independence Art Press
419 Janisch Road, Houston, Texas 77018
www.independenceartpress.com

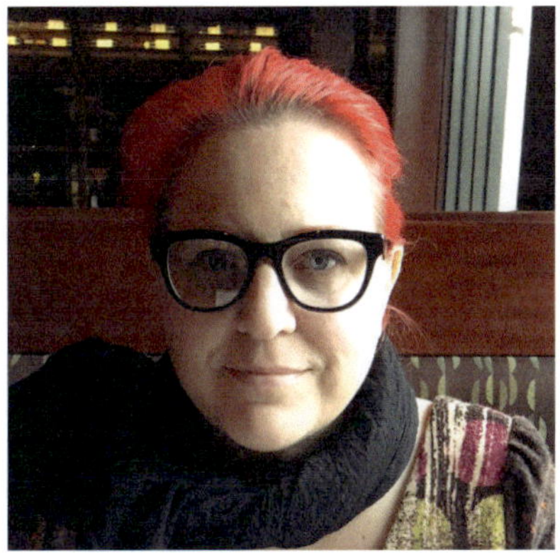

Thank you to all the friends, family, doctors, nurses, dogs, cats, chickens, bartenders and complete strangers who helped me get through this shitstorm of a year.

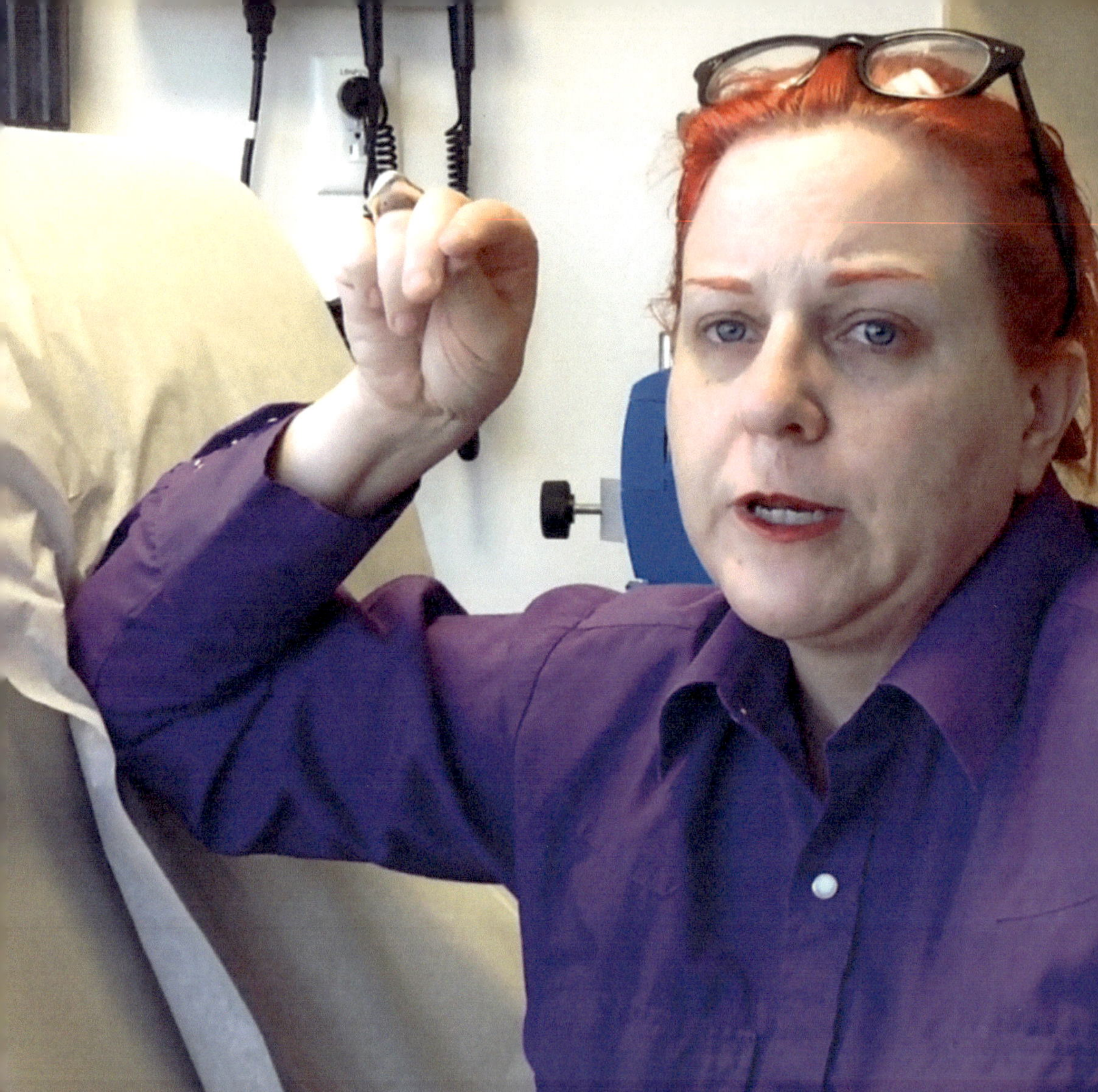

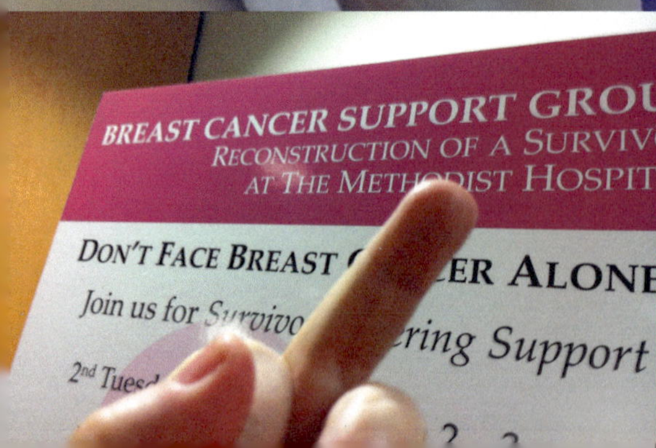
BREAST CANCER SUPPORT
RECONSTRUCTION OF A
AT THE METHODIST
DON'T FACE BREAST
Join us for

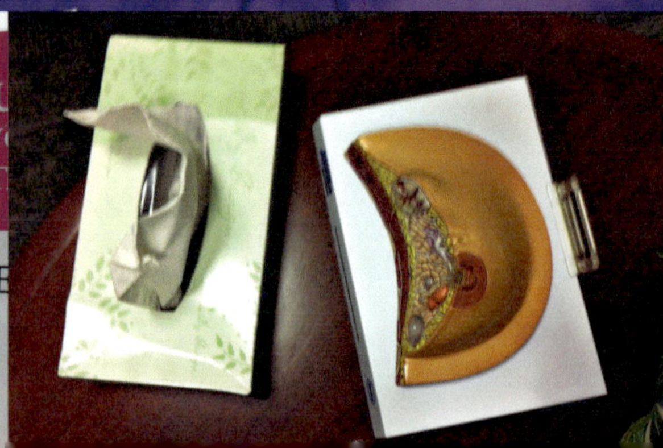

December 14, 2013

It's amazing how things can change.

Yesterday morning, I was getting ready to donate a kidney. I had been through test after test, waiting for the donation chain to come together. There was one final request from the clinic that was to receive my kidney — for a mammogram. I hadn't had one for years, so the hospital arranged one on short notice.

I'm not giving a kidney anymore because I have (what appears at this point to be) ductal carcinoma in-situ aka "stage zero" breast cancer. We'll do a biopsy in a few weeks and then figure out what to do, but my expectation is that I will be getting a complete boob job pretty soon. I feel really sad that I can't donate, and that I broke the chain that would have helped so many people. I hope they can put it back together soon.

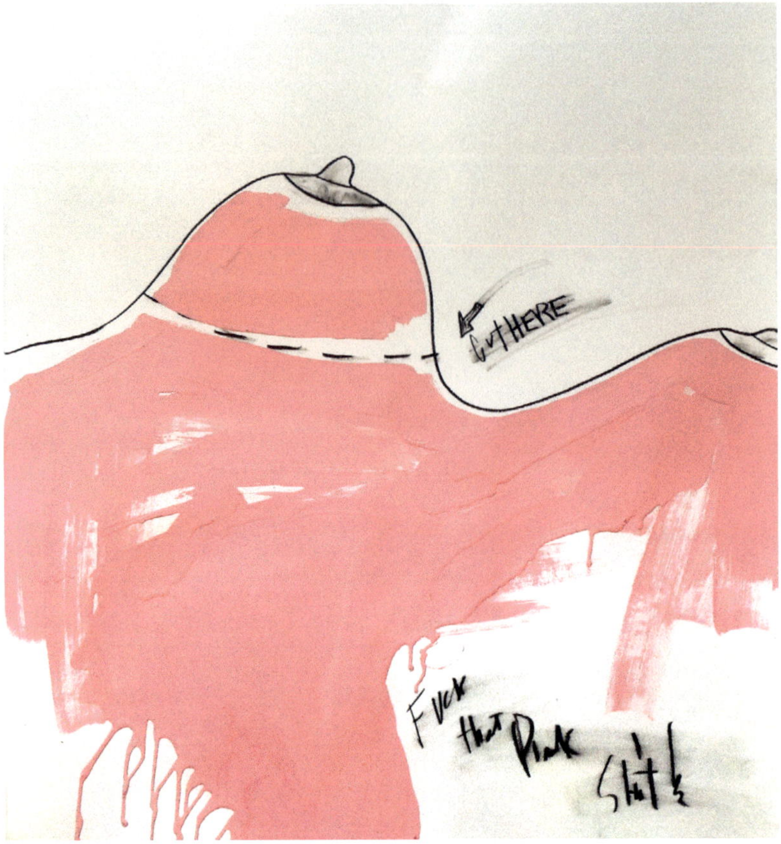

Cut Here
2014, 24" x 24"
Acrylic and charcoal on paper

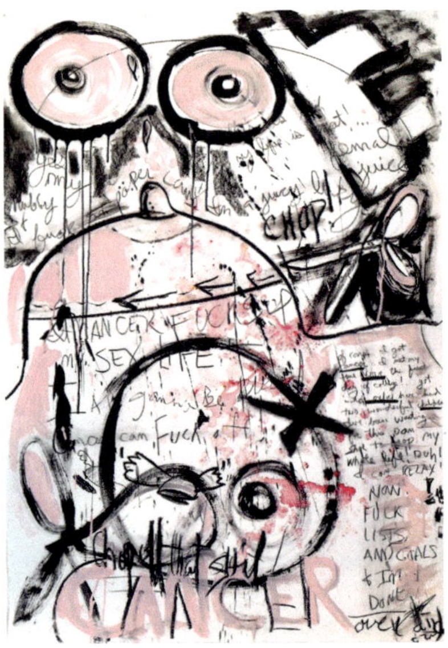

Chop
2014, 36" x 48"
Acrylic, charcoal
and pencil on paper

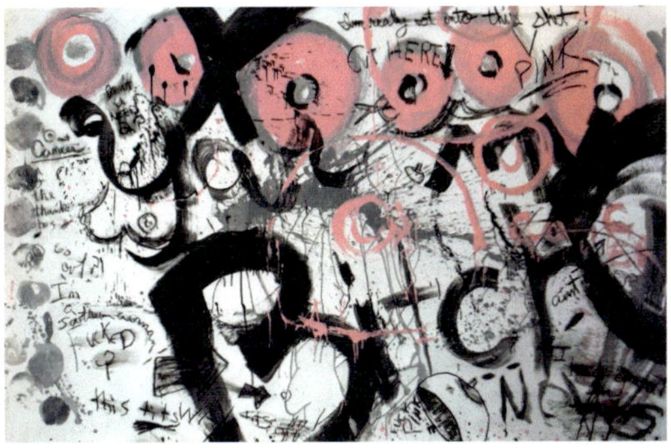

Bitch
2014, 180" x 120"
Acrylic, charcoal
and pencil on paper

Studio, 2014
Photo: Jan Johnson

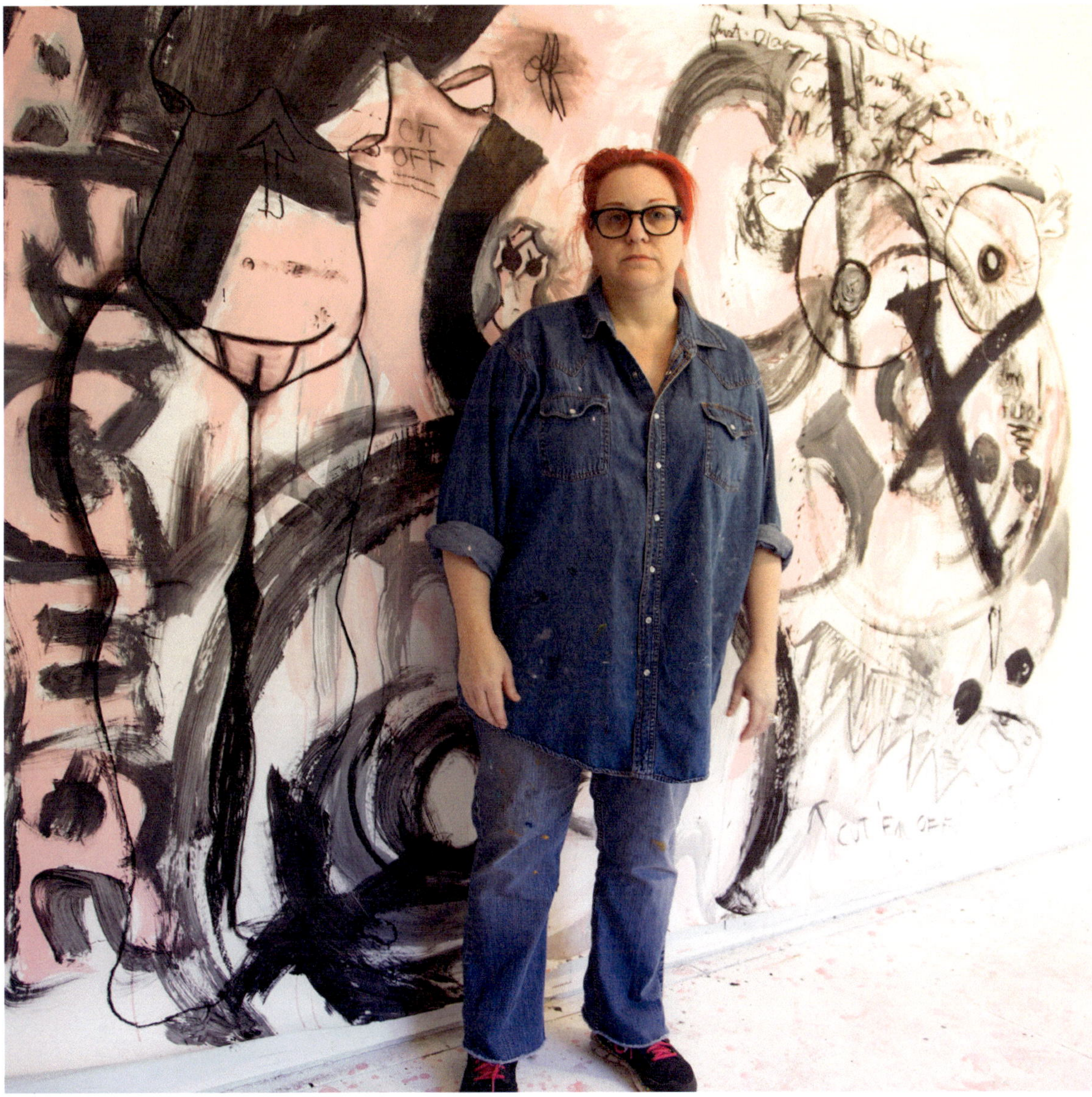

I have a bit more information about my boobies based on last week's biopsy.

It appears that the initial thinking — that it is DCIS — is correct. There is also a small spot of an invasive cancer, but the fact that it is there does not change the treatment plan. Next step is to meet with the plastic surgeon and to do the BRCA genetic test. Once we have that result, we'll meet with the medical oncologist.

It sounds like surgery is several weeks away at the soonest, but there is not a firm schedule yet. I feel better now that we seem to be moving forward with a plan. It's all very Angelina Jolie. Rock on!

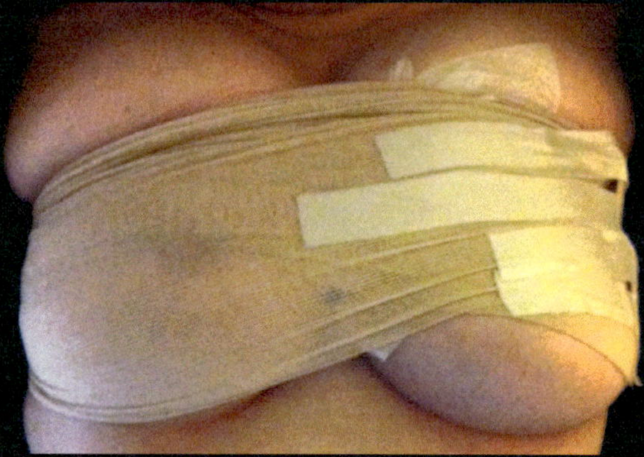

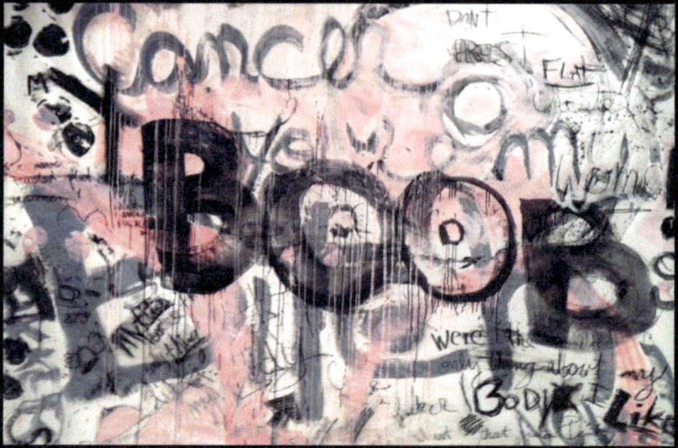

Cancer Took My Boobs
2014, 180"x 120"
Acrylic and charcoal on paper

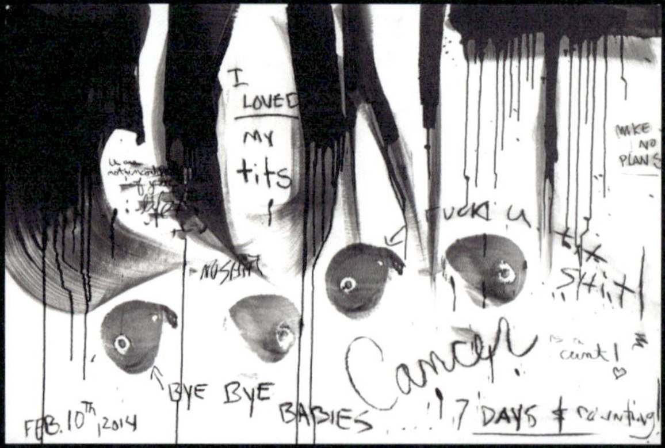

Cancer is a Cunt
2014, 36"x 24"

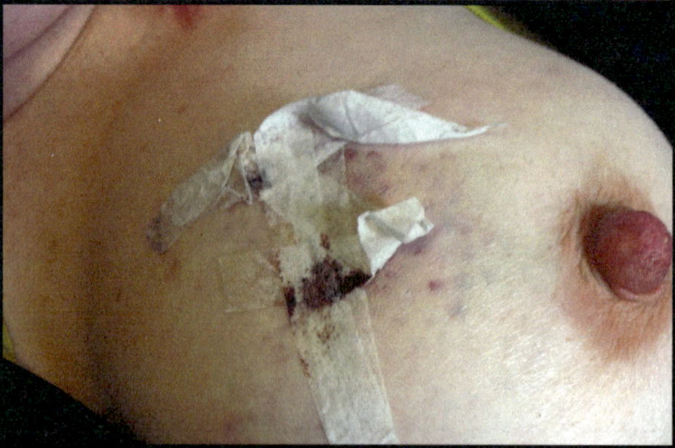

Biopsy Photos
Photos: Everett Taasevigen

Met with the oncologist today who had more info from the biopsy last week.

New diagnosis is "invasive ductal carcinoma." Again, the invasive part does not really change the treatment plan compared to "ductal carcinoma in situ." The difference is that some of the naughty little cells have escaped their cozy ductal home. There is no evidence that any of them have made it to a lymph node yet (which is good.) This is one of the things we will find out during surgery and in the week or so after.

Apparently us breast cancer patients are lucky because research has figured out how to identify different types of breast cancers. Mine is being stimulated by estrogen & progesterone. This is also good because there are medications that interfere with this mechanism. My cancer is also a very slow-growing type. I'm not likely to need chemo or radiation.

In any case, the left one is a goner. It will mostly be up to me whether or not to have a matching set installed. In most cases, the reconstruction procedure occurs several weeks or months after the mastectomy procedure, so that if they need to do something else to get the cancer they don't ruin the brand new tits.

Shocking fact: one in eight women will be diagnosed with breast cancer. About 90% of those are from complete randomness. The other 10% are hereditary cases where both the BRCA1 and BRCA2 genes are malfunctioning. We do not yet have my BRCA genetic test results back, but I am likely negative.

Everyone please go have your tits squeezed by a professional for me. (And then later by someone you like!)

Ending with a quote from my good friend BMoody: "This is all such a fucking bore!"

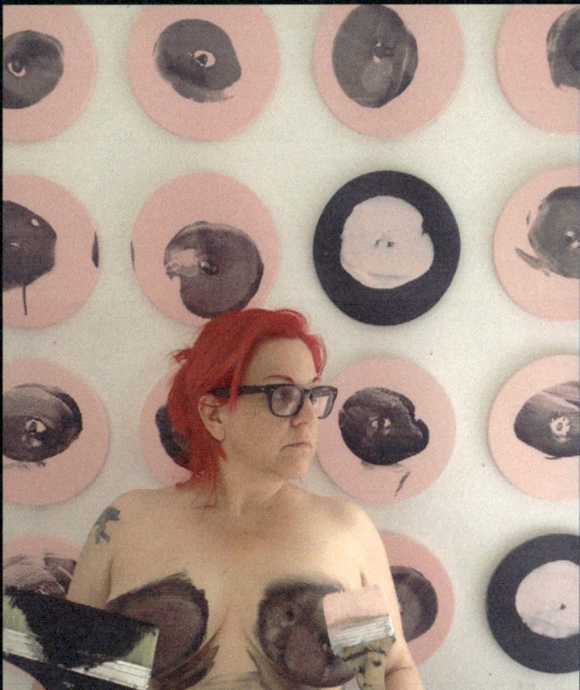

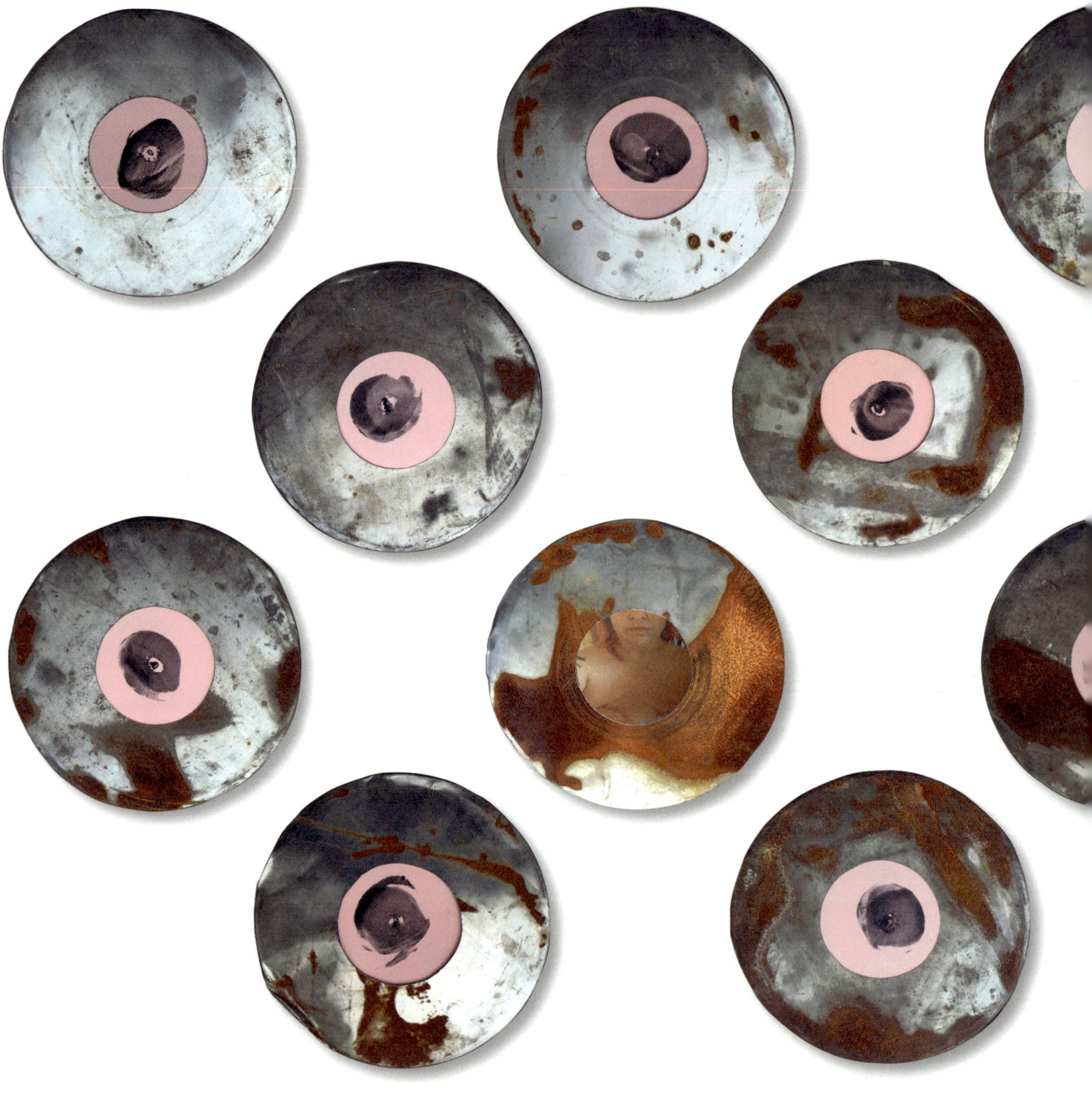

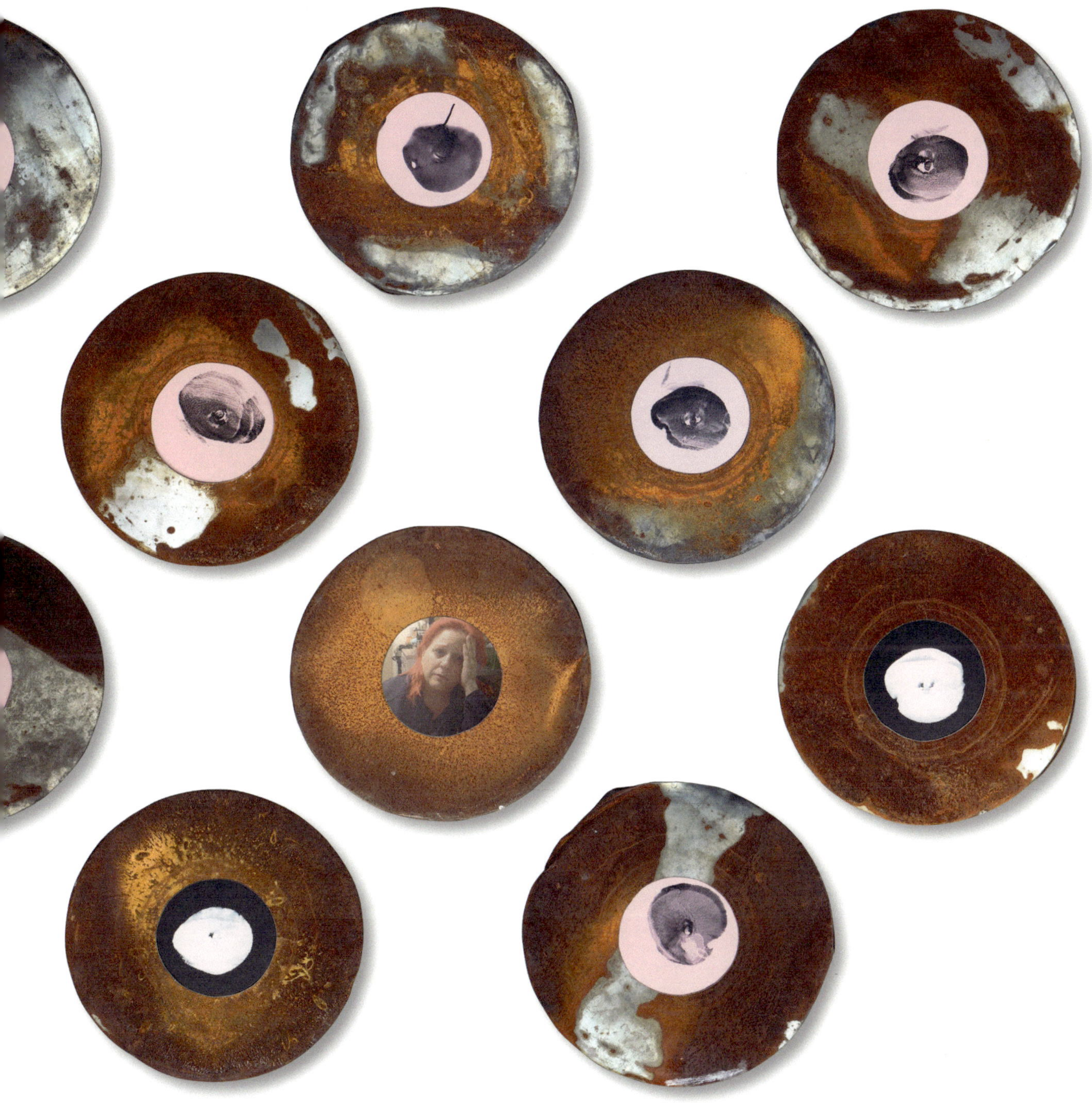

One in Eight
2015, dimensions variable,
24" diameter each
Breast prints in acrylic on canvas,
barrel tops, video interviews

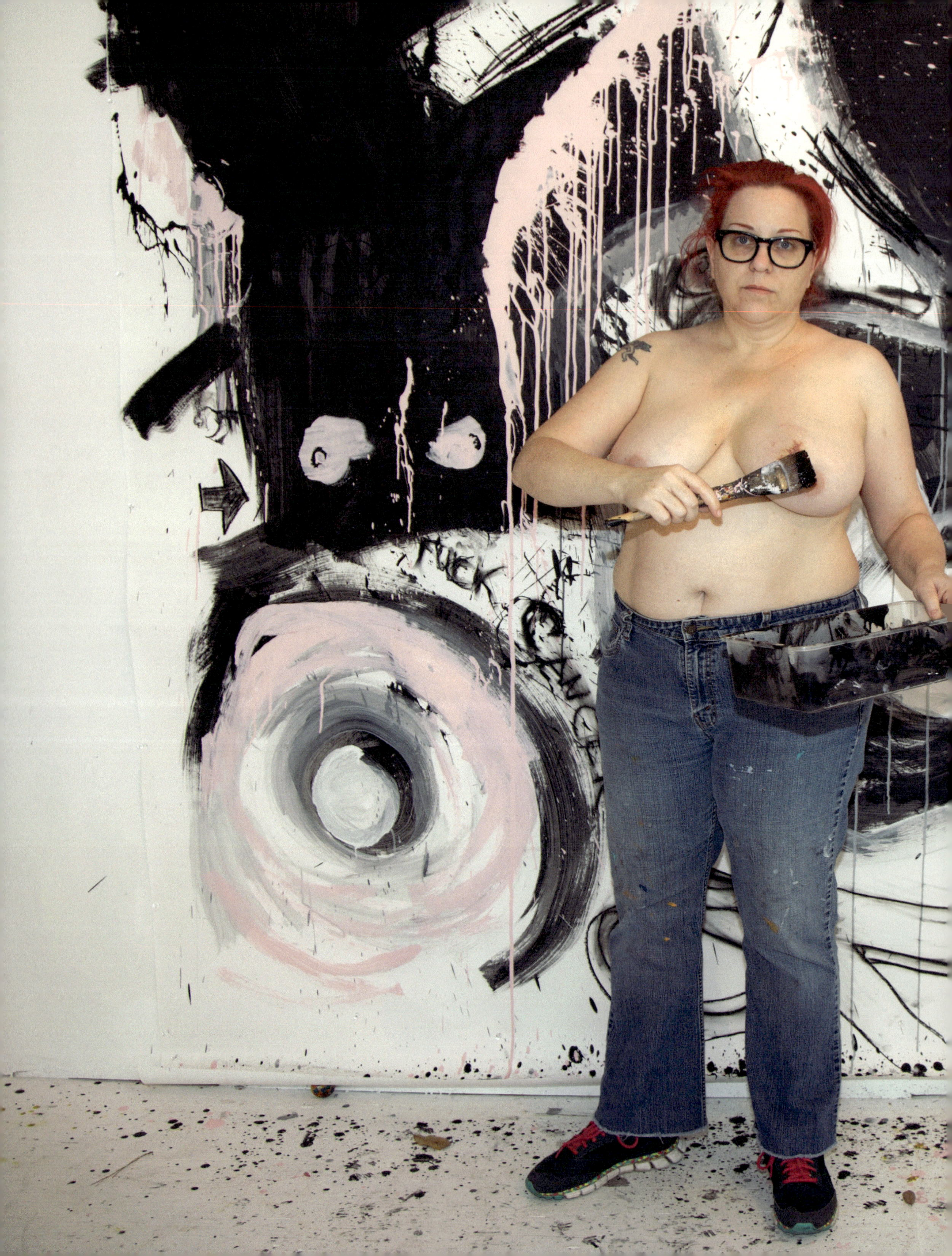
FUCK

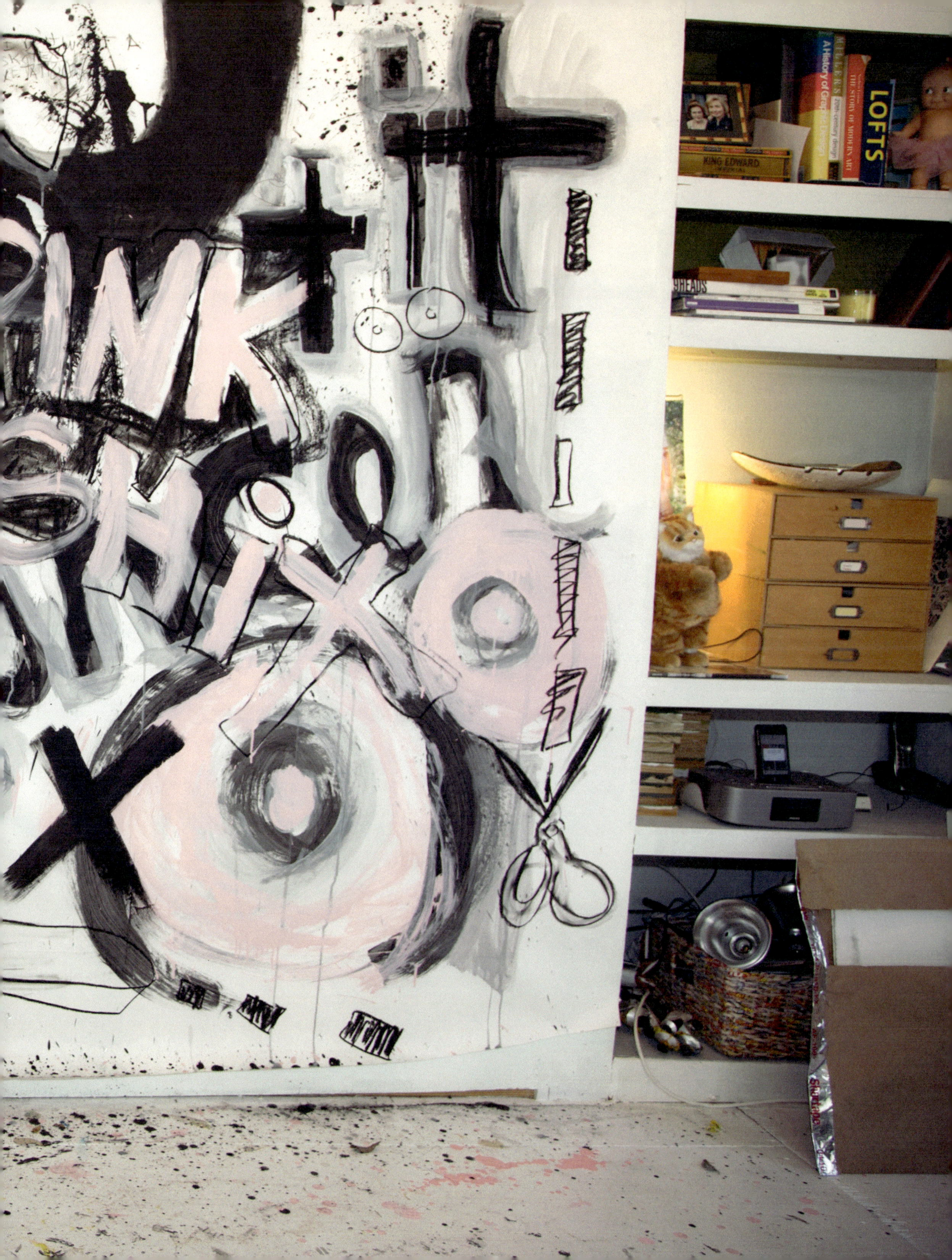
KING EDWARD
LOFTS

January 22, 2014

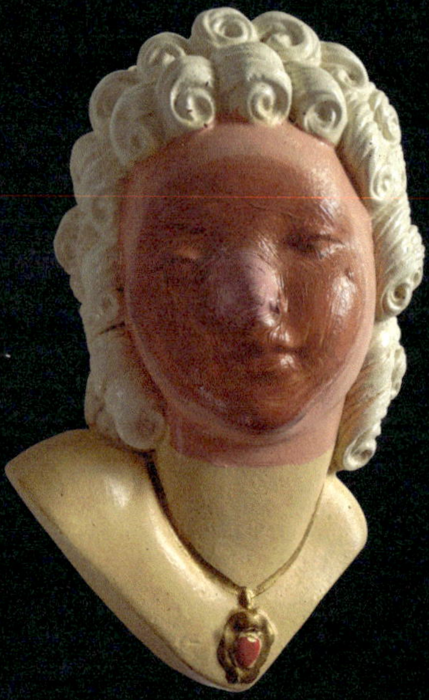

Boob Head
2014, 6" x 8" x 3"
Oil on porcelain

Met with plastic surgeon today. I decided to do both to keep things symmetrical. Surgery likely in about a month. During the mastectomy surgery, he will put "expanders" under the pectoral muscles. A few weeks later, these can gradually be inflated until they get to the size I want (not very big.) Then comes another, smaller surgery to remove the expanders and install the final implants. Decoration (nipple tattoos etc) will be sorted out after all that is done.

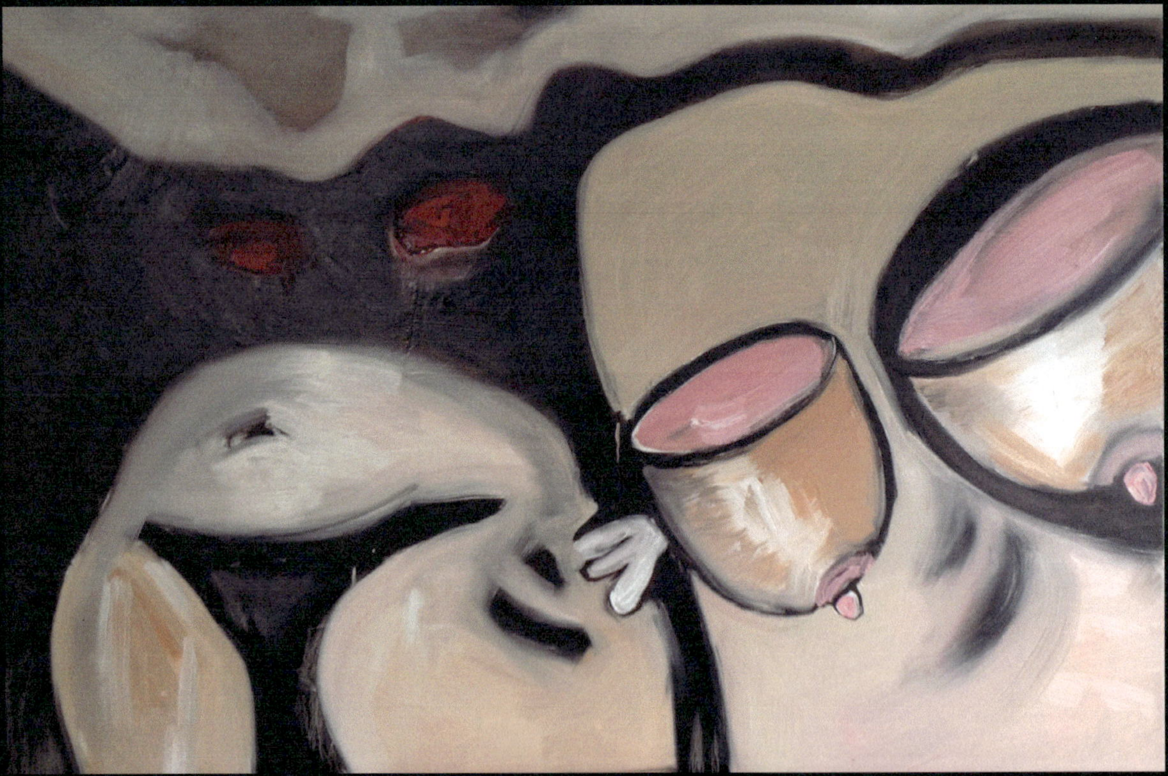

Flying Tits
2014, 72" x 48"
Oil on canvas

had a consultation with the genetic counselor last week. I already had the BRC-A and BRC-B test (both negative), but they really want to figure out why my body manifested so much cancer, seemingly out of nowhere.

There are additional genetic tests which they would like to do. While a positive BRC-A test explains about 10% of all breast cancers, these other tests have much smaller predictive abilities.

I guess genetic counseling is required because these tests can tell you things that you and your family might not want to hear or know. These issues are not very important to me because a) I already had breast cancer, and b) I only gave birth to males. I agreed to the tests because they won't cost me anything more (we have already maxed out our annual deductible) and maybe my results will help with the scientific research.

We also met with Dr. Rodriguez, the oncologist. He had results back from the genetic type tests on some of my tumors. The question, in my case, is whether all of the cancers found are of the same type. If they are all the same, non-aggressive types, then further treatments are not necessary. The first two tumors they tested (the two largest ones) were the same -- not aggressive. They are testing a few more now and we'll get those results back in a few weeks.

The guidance, therefore, is not to prescribe chemotherapy or radiation therapy, since neither improves the final outcome any more than doing nothing. I was very happy to hear this.

He will prescribe Tamoxifen, a drug that blocks the female hormones progesterone and estrogen. Those hormones were spurring my cancers to grow, and blocking them will shut down that mechanism. There are potentially side-effects, including the early and sudden onset of menopause. I had a hysterectomy a few years ago and there was some confusion afterwards whether or not the ovaries were taken out too. I need to find out if I still have ovaries because that will make a big difference. Stephen is looking for his snorkel.

Fuck This Pink Shi
2014, 180" x 120"
Acrylic and charcoal on pape

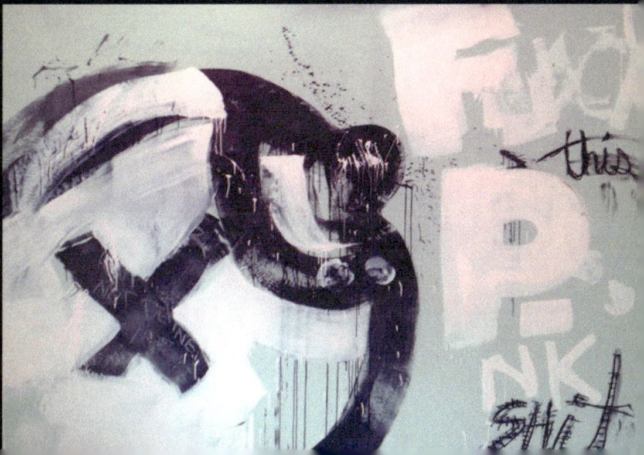

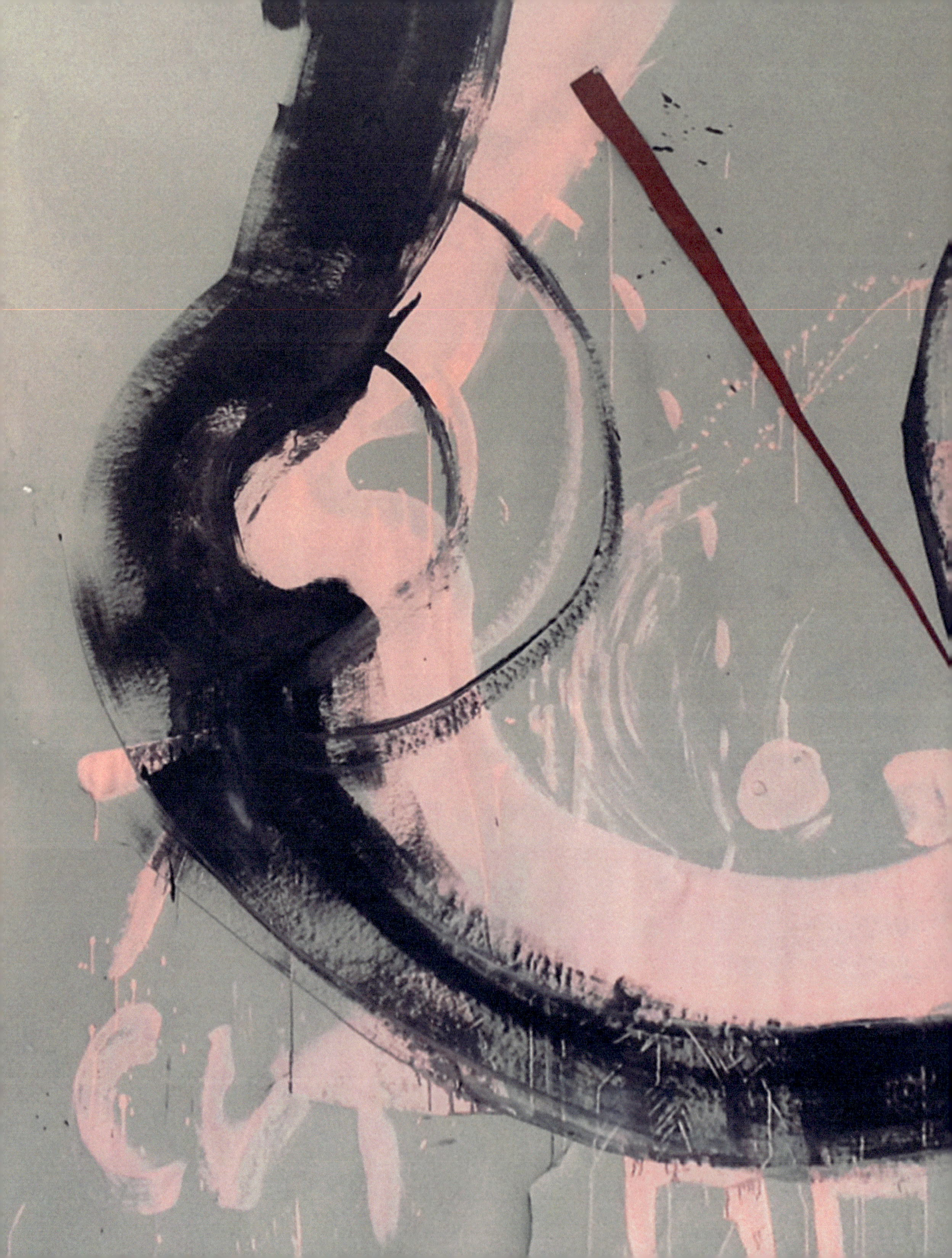

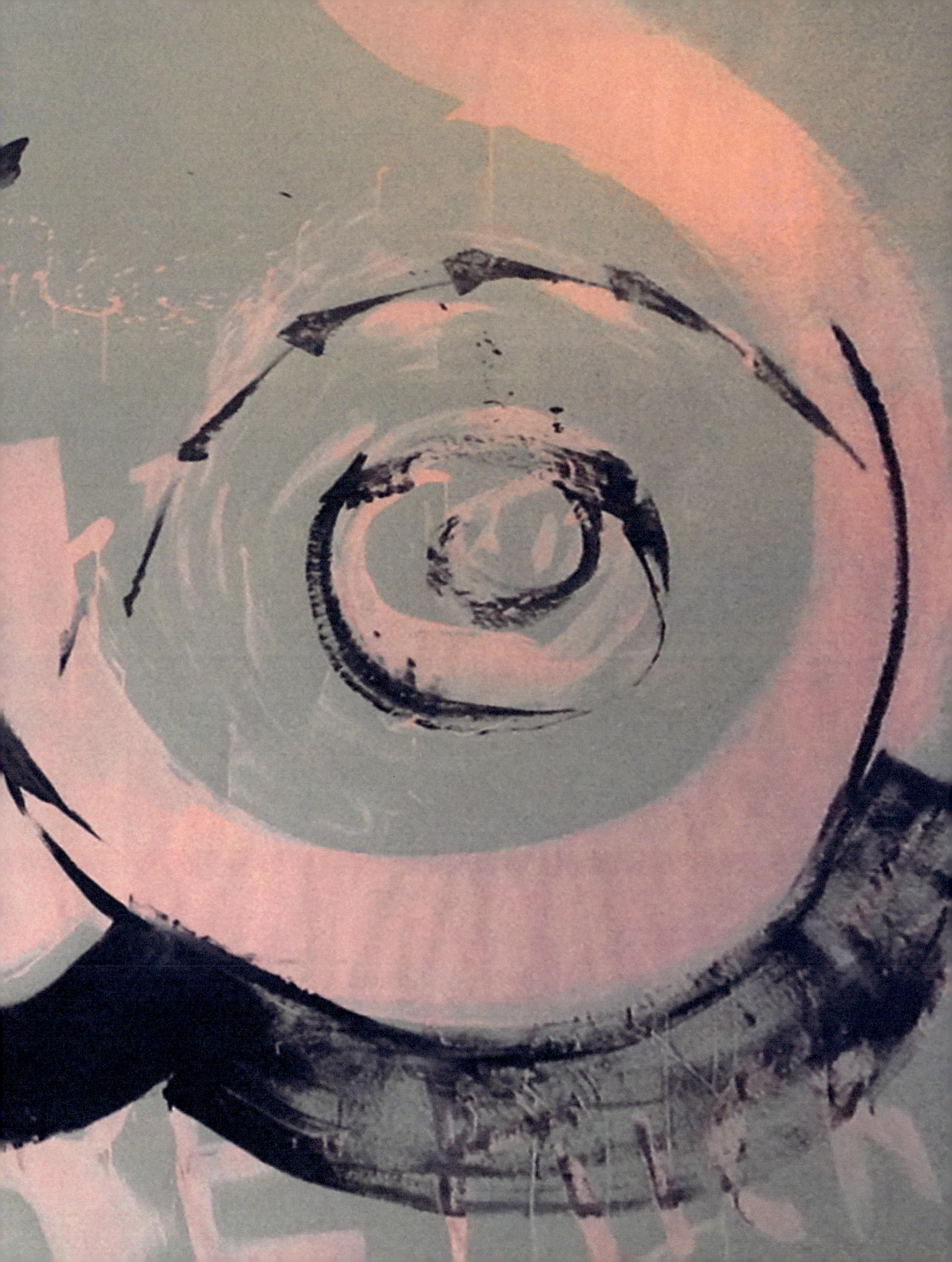

Previous pages
Cut Here
2014, 120" x 80"
Acrylic on paper

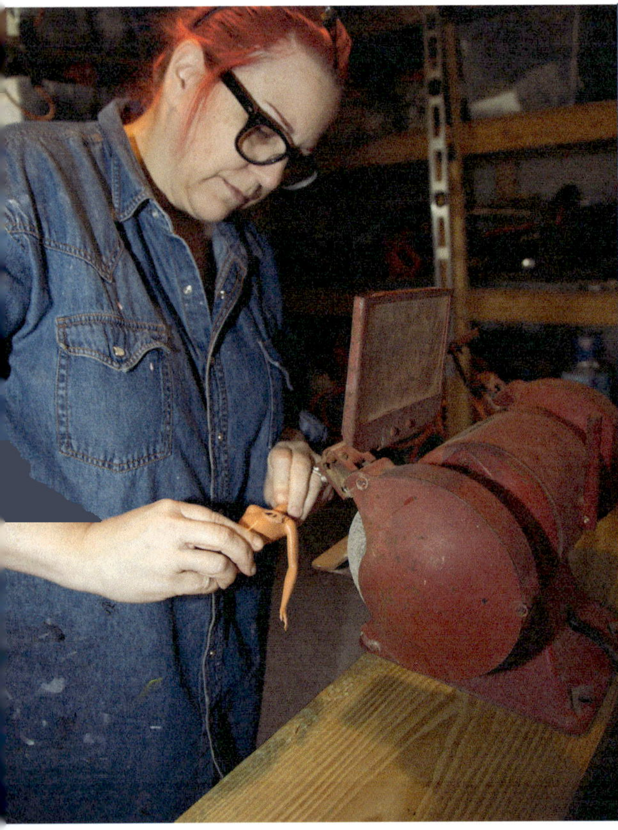

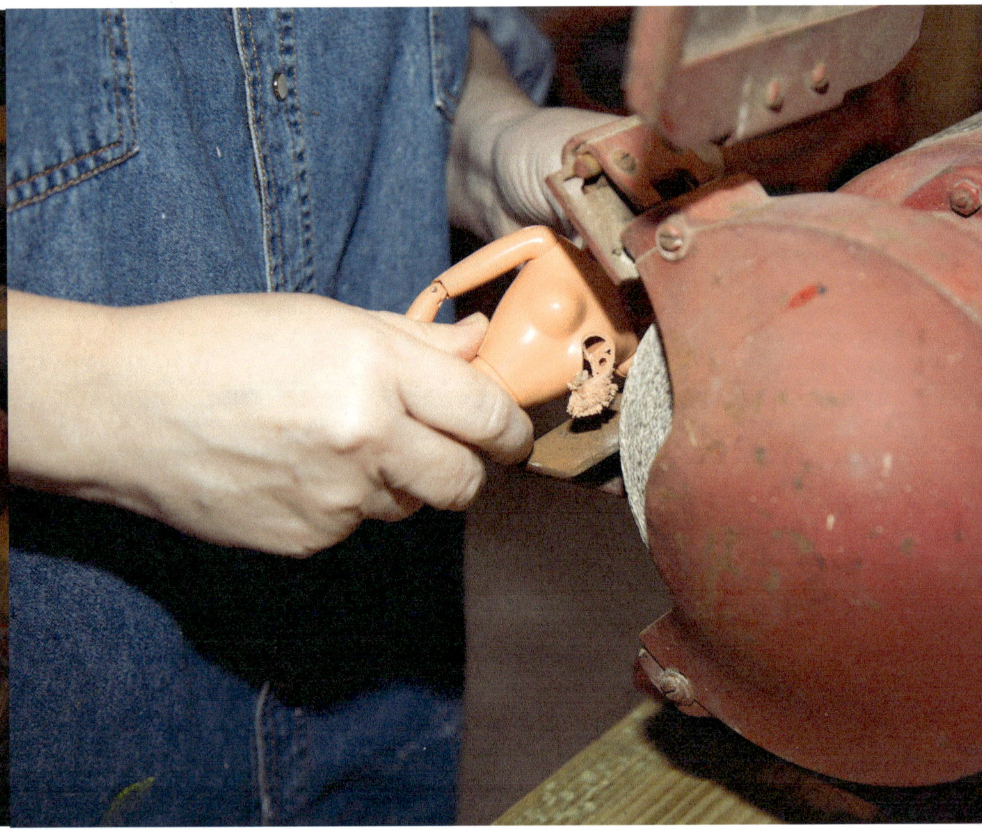

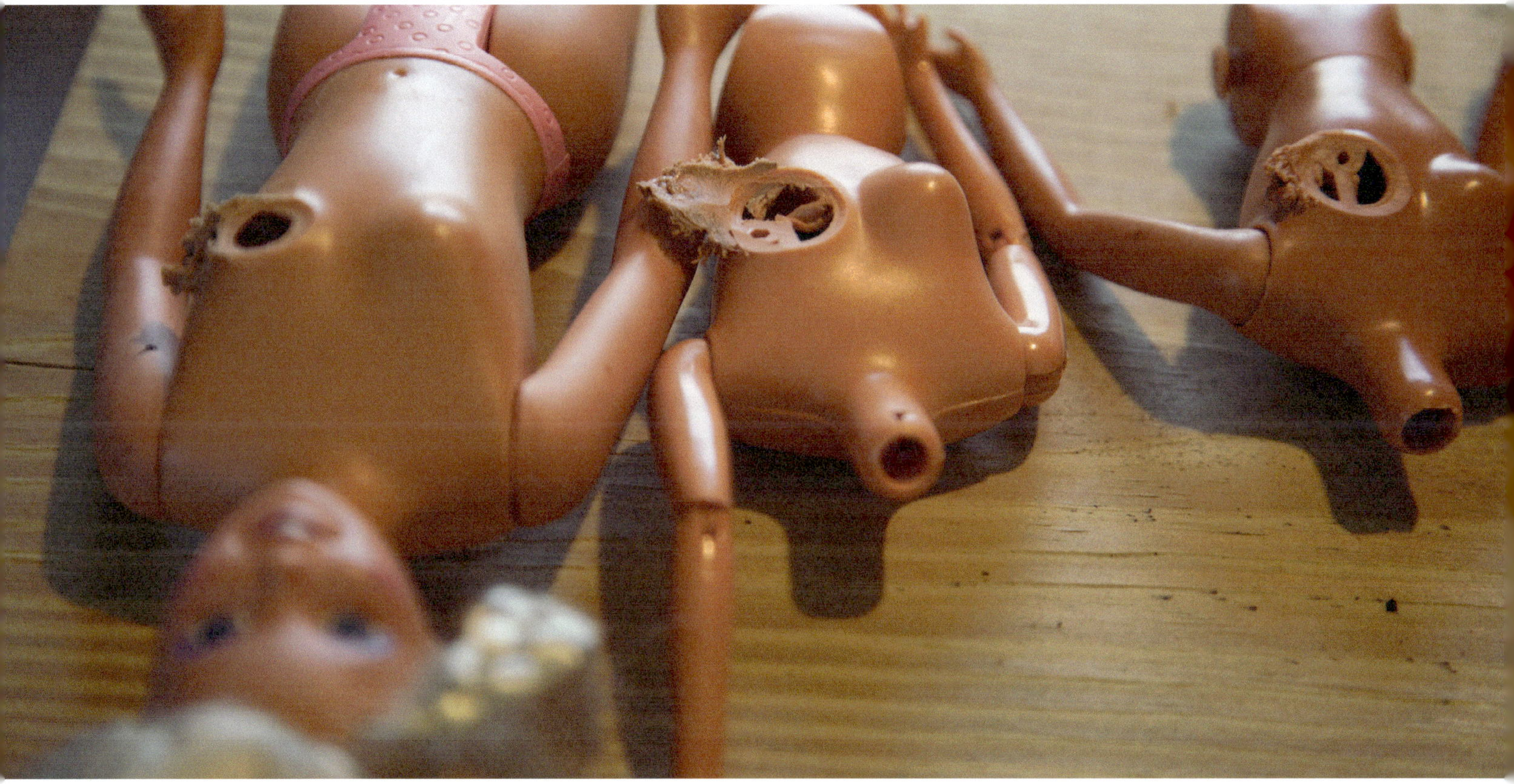

Barbie Grinding
2014
Performance with Barbie dolls and
my grandfather's motorized grinder
Photos and video: Jan Johnson

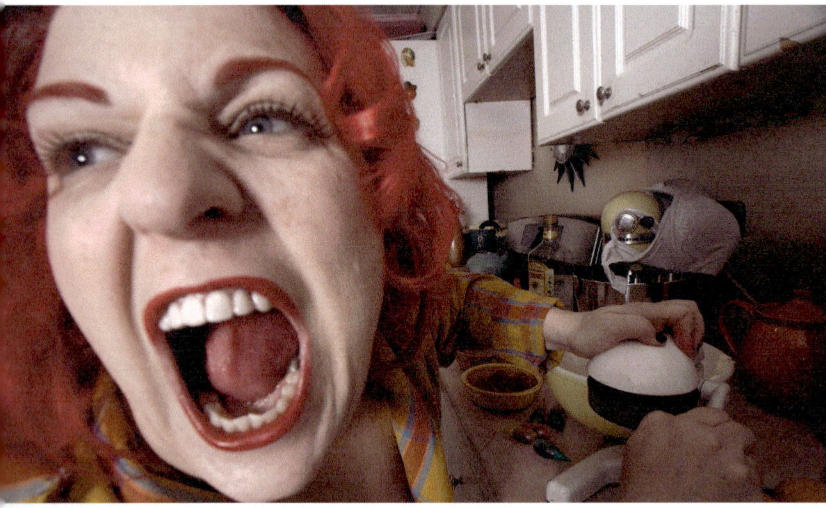
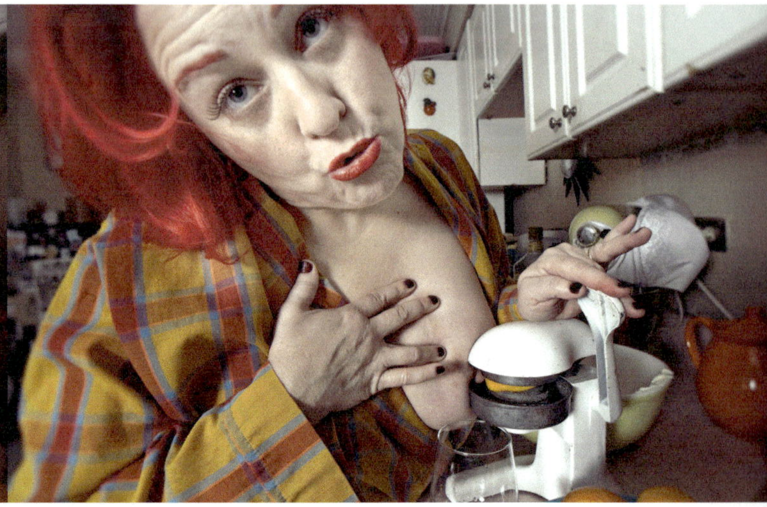
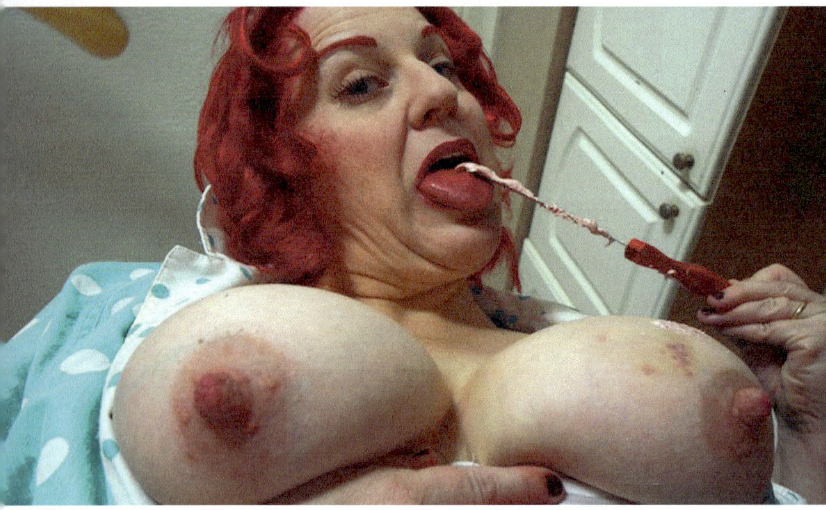
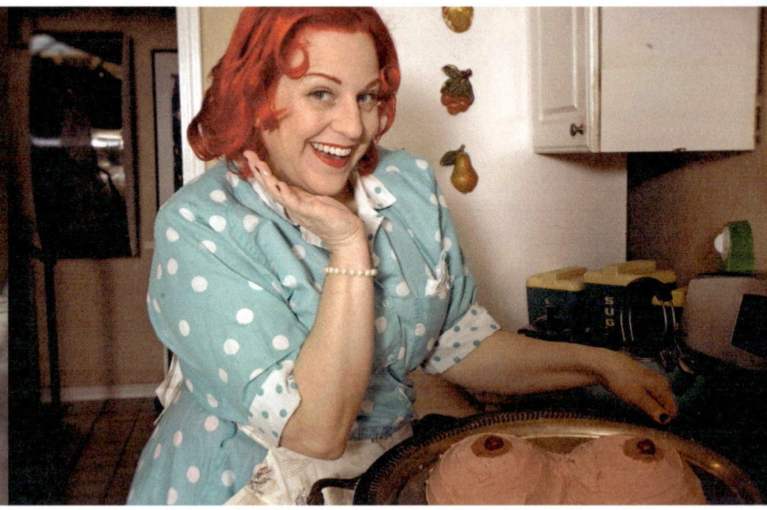

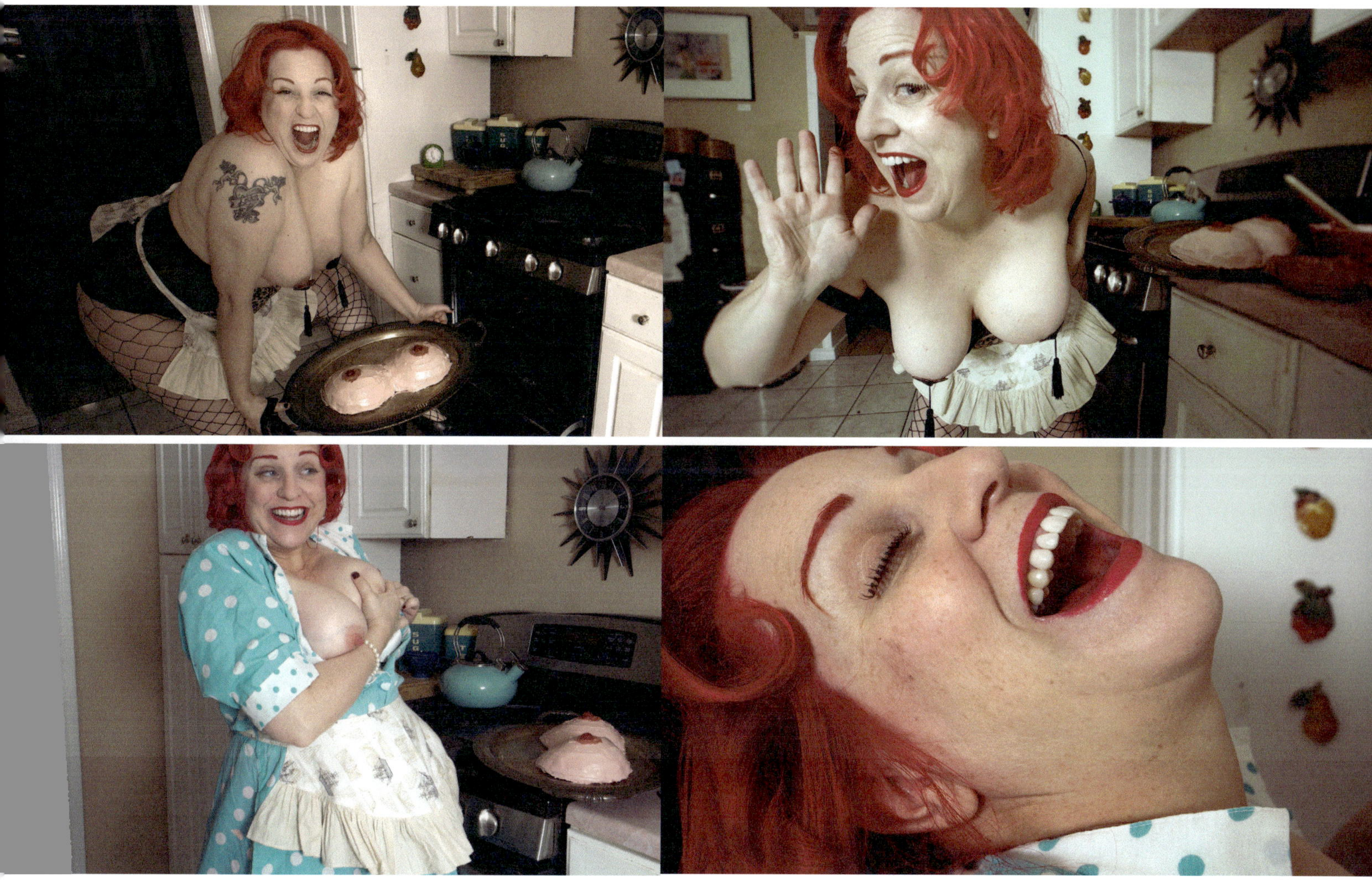

Kitchen Performance
2014
Photos: Everett Taasevigen

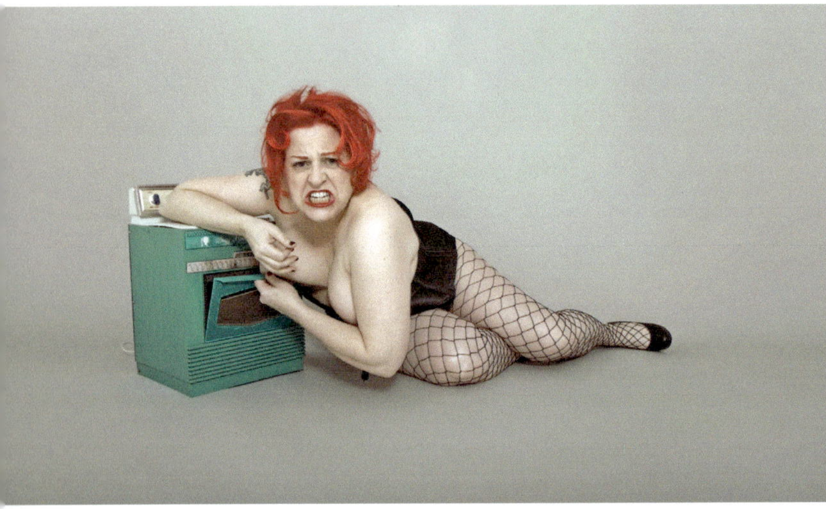
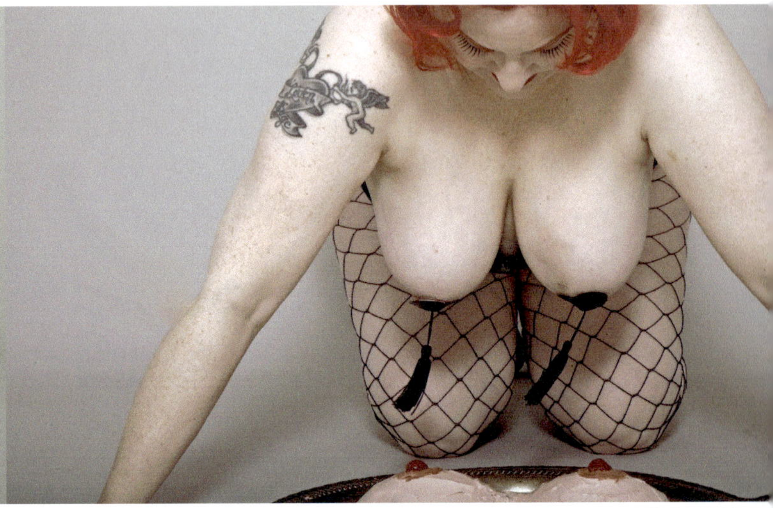
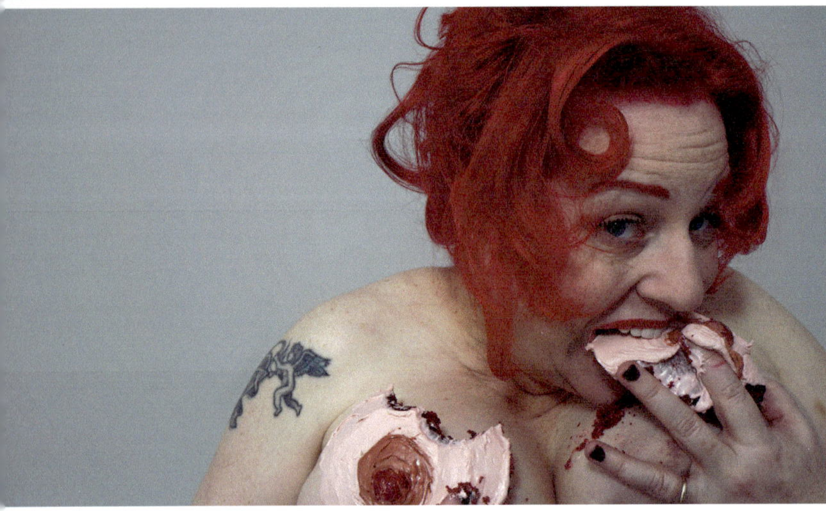
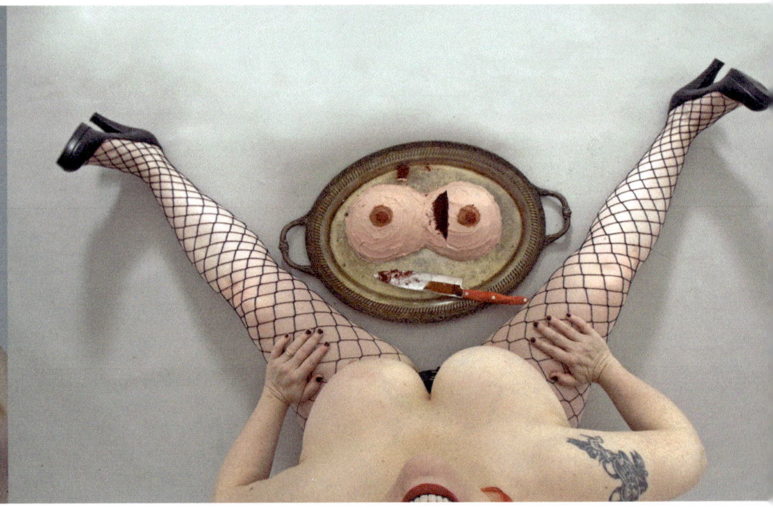

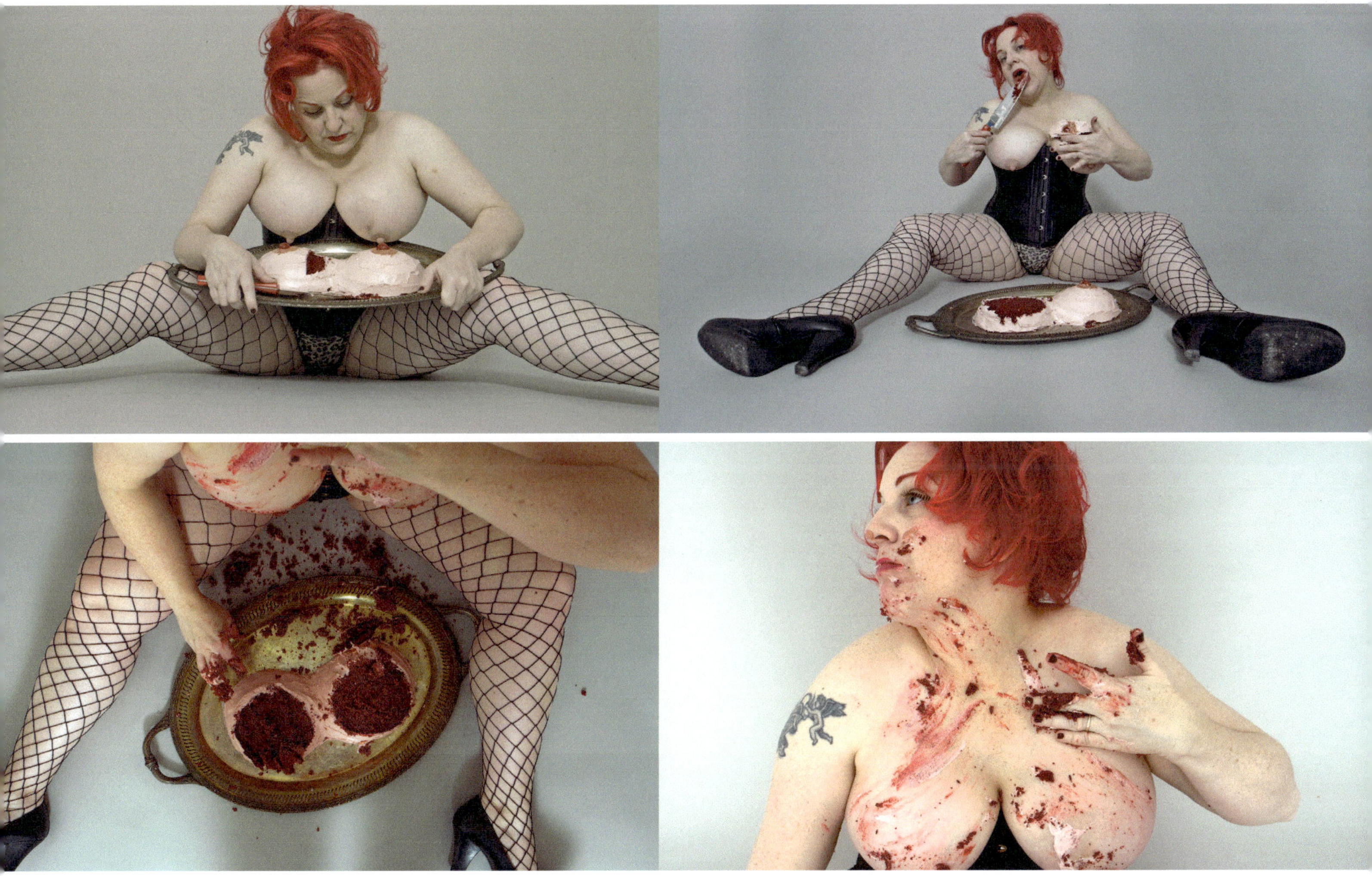

Kitchen Performance
2014
Photos: Everett Taasevigen

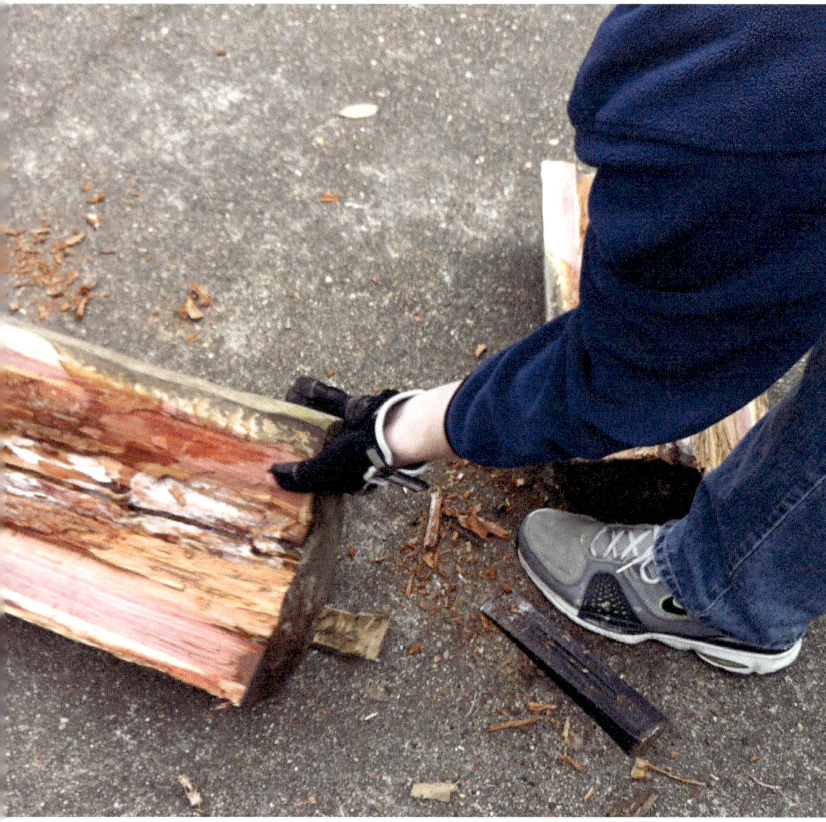
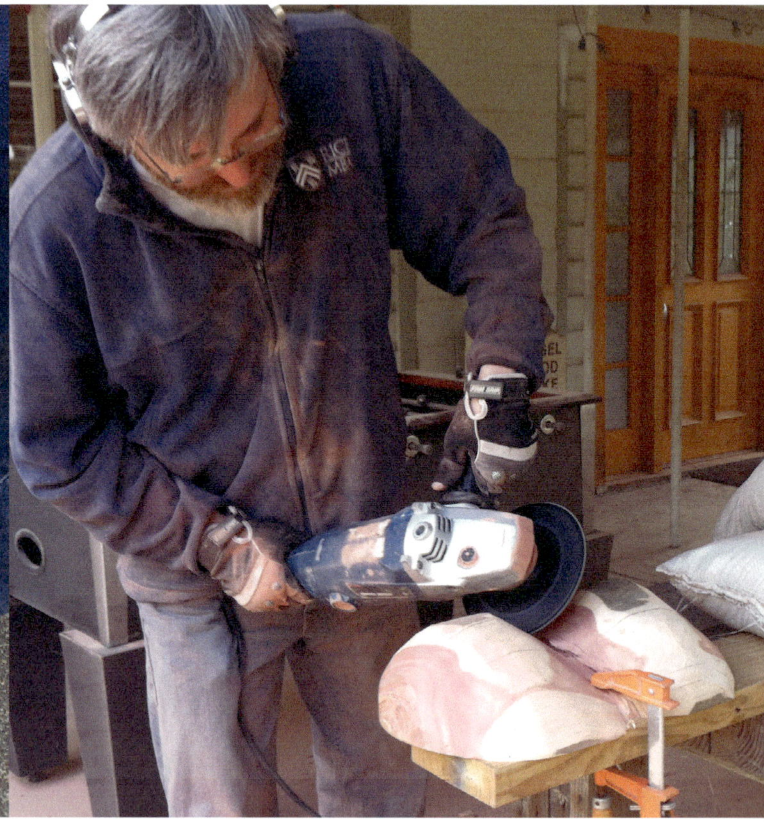

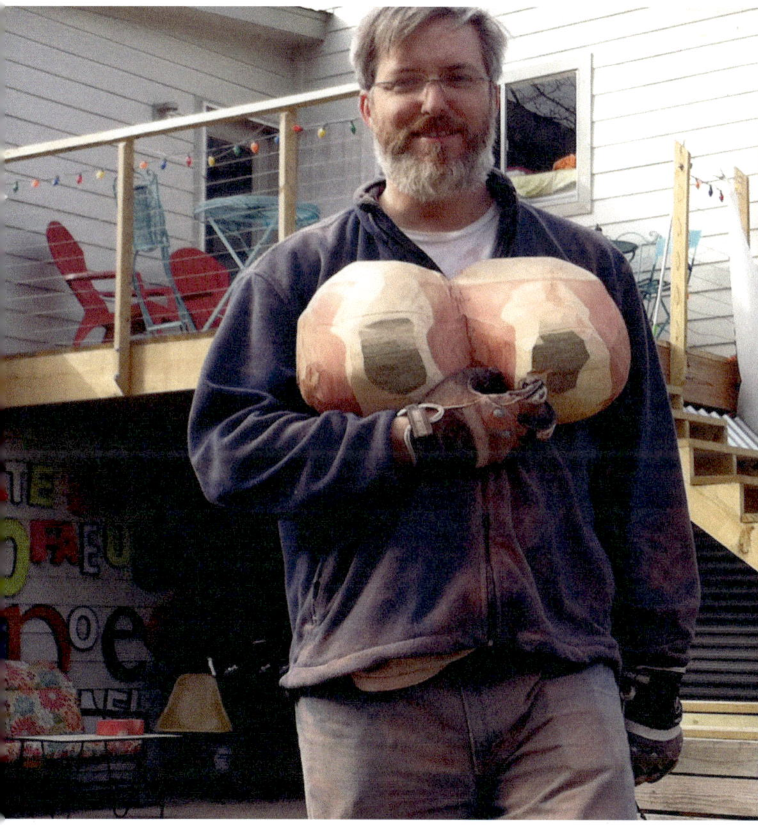

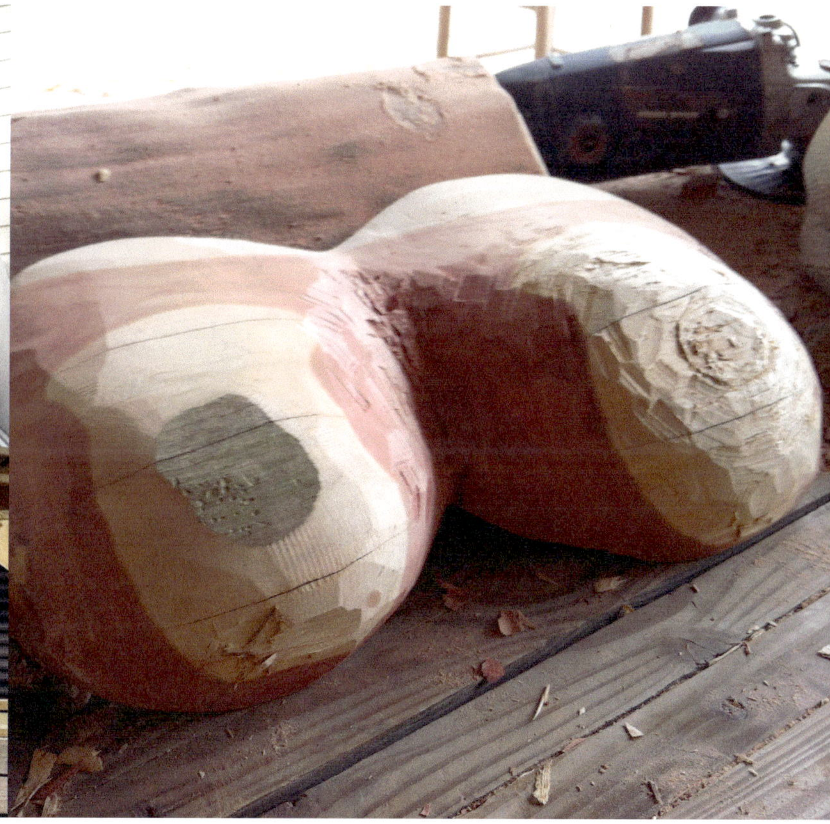

Coping Skills
2014
Performance, cedar log
The day before my mastectomy, I sat by the fire drinking wine while Stephen shaped a stump from our yard into a set of boobs. Every few minutes he would come over with calipers and ask me to lift up my shirt. Thouroughly fun day.

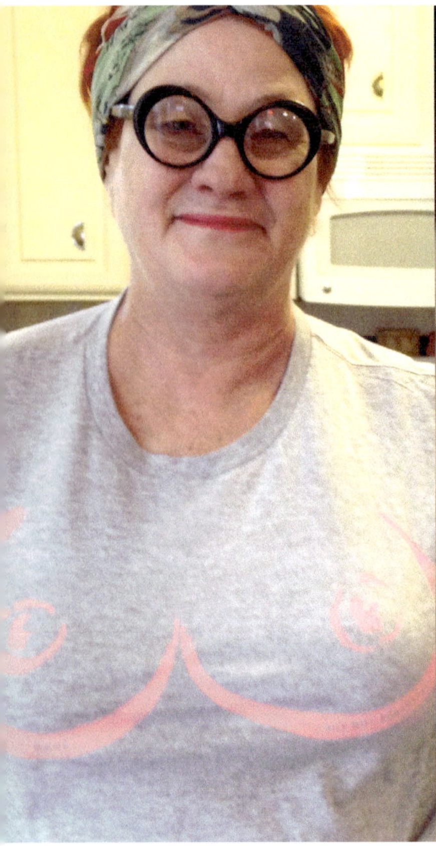
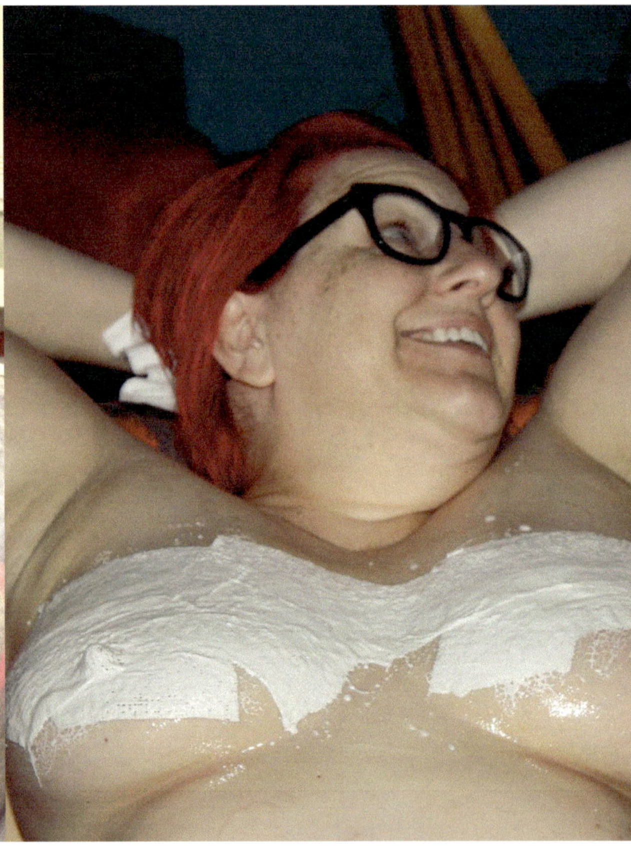
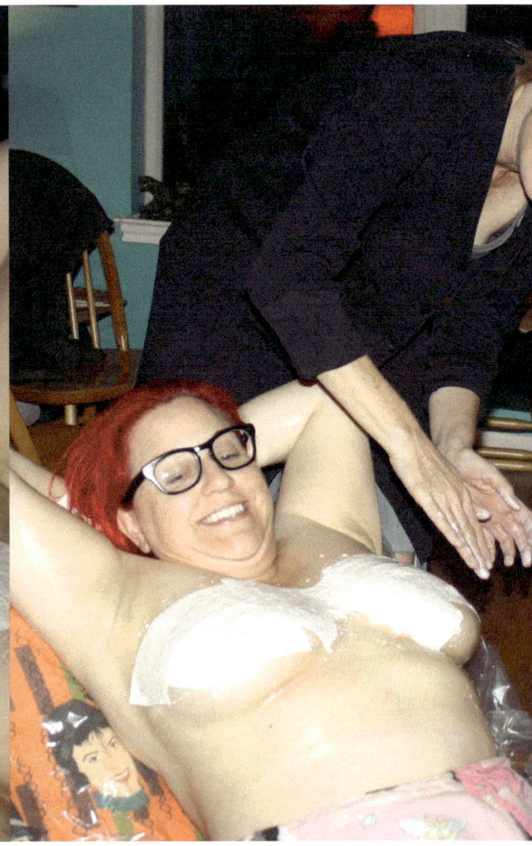

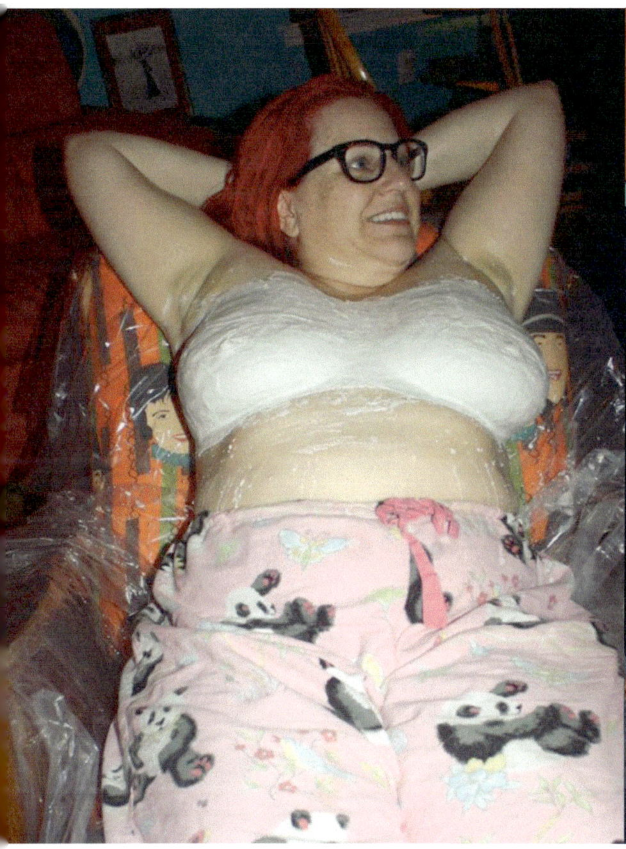

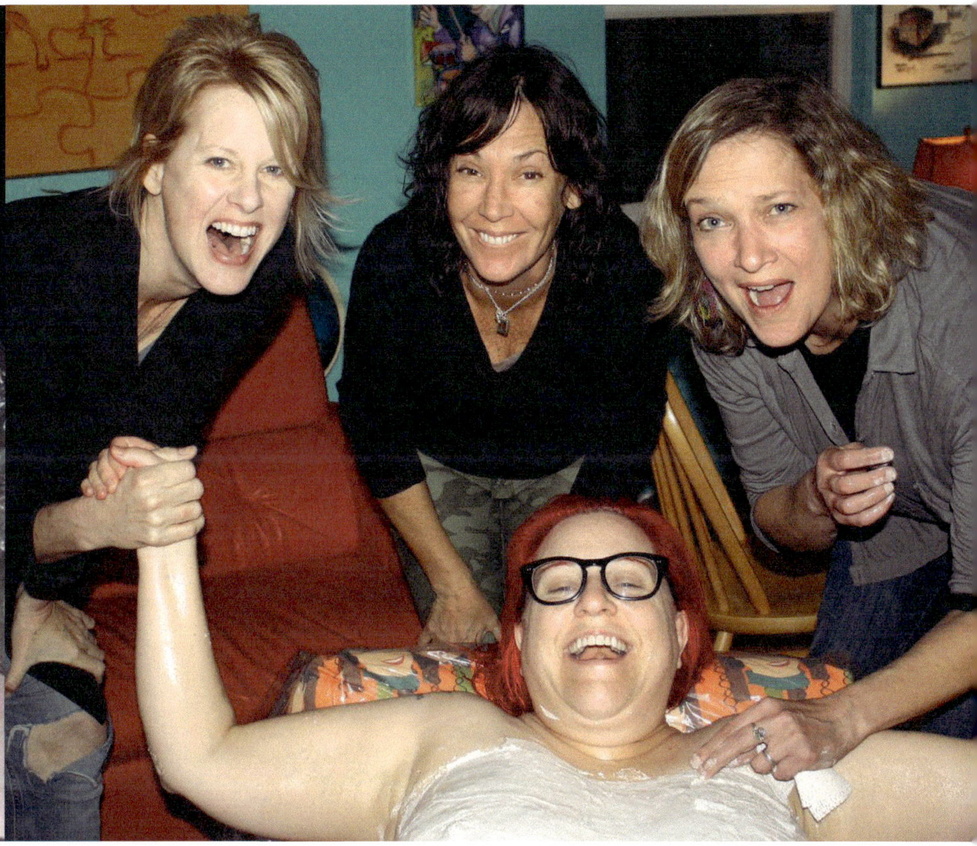

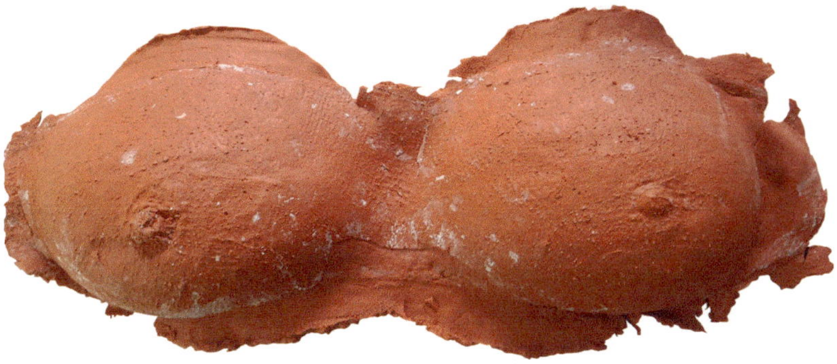

Austin Boob Casting Party
2014
Surround yourself with a supportive tribe because when the shit hits the fan, you are going to need them.

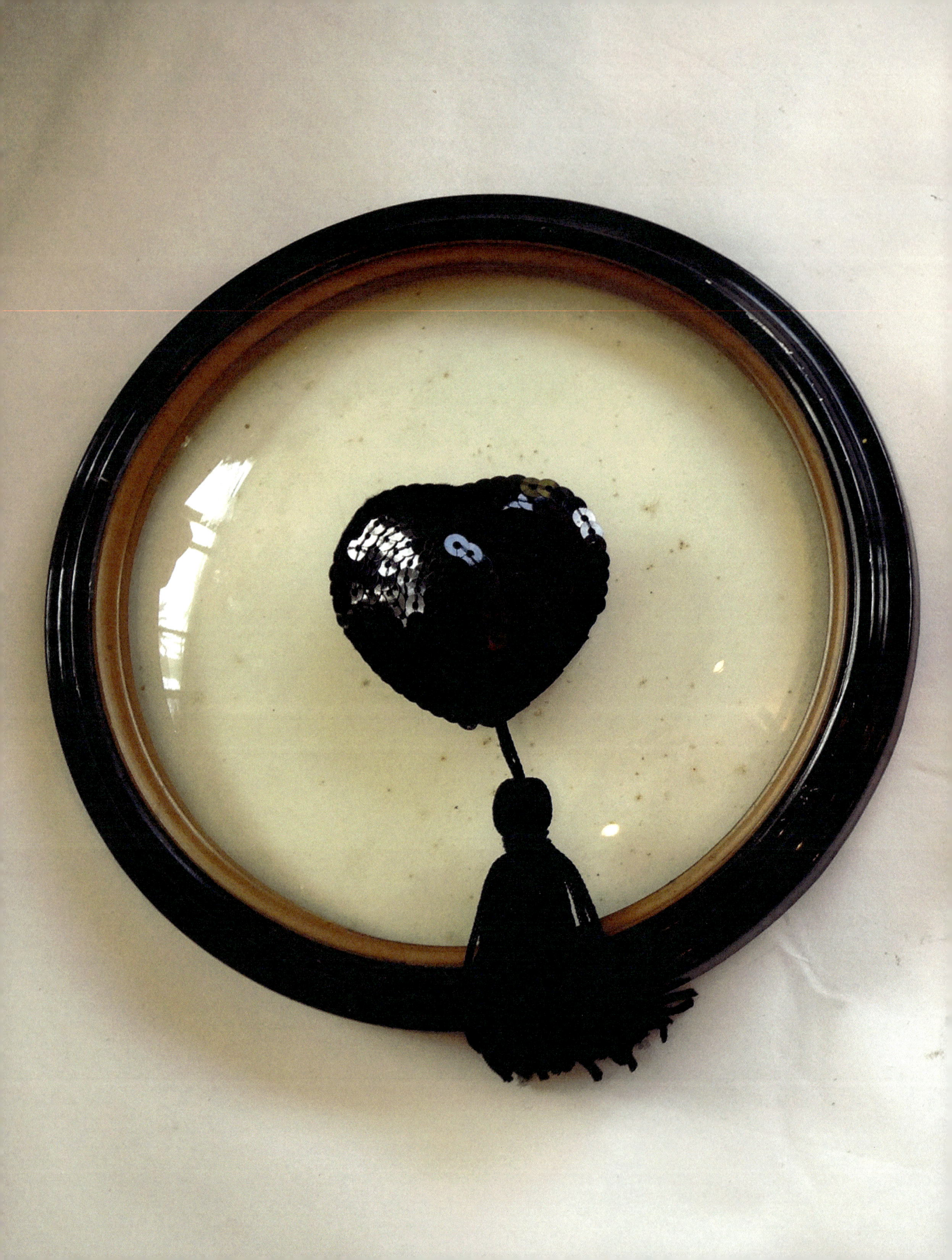

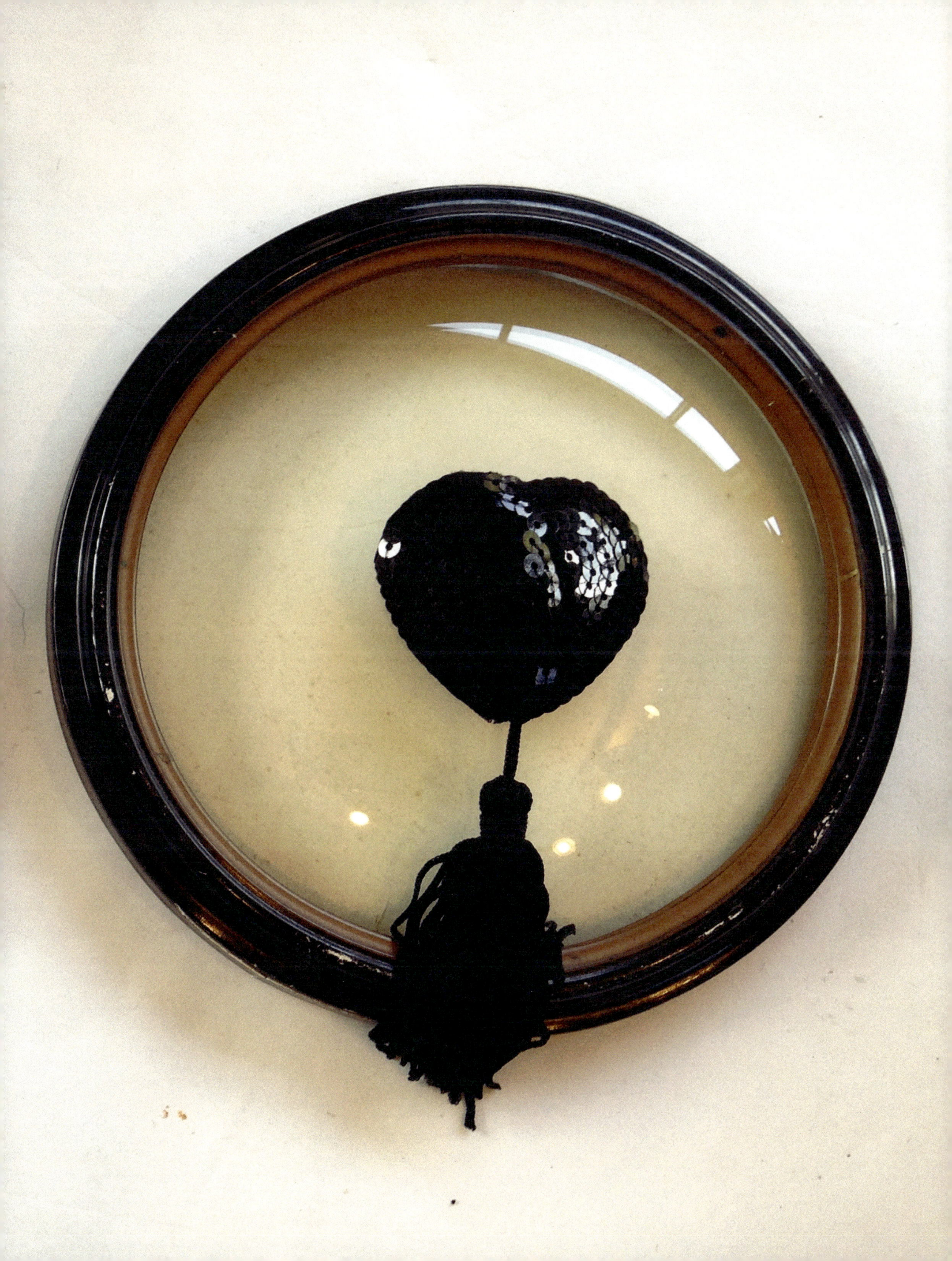

Previous pages
Preserved
2015, 16"x 7"
Pasties on Victorian glass frames

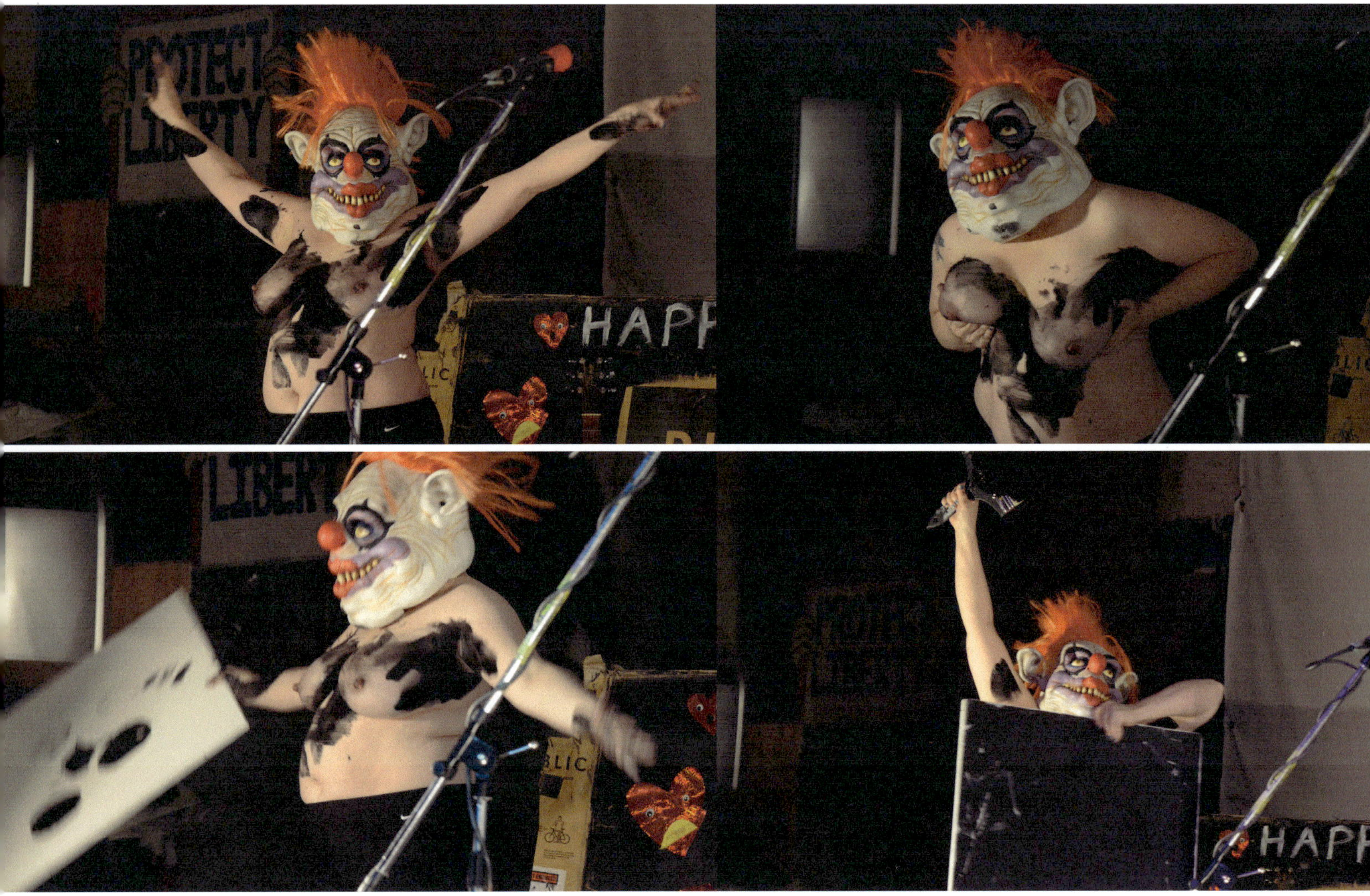

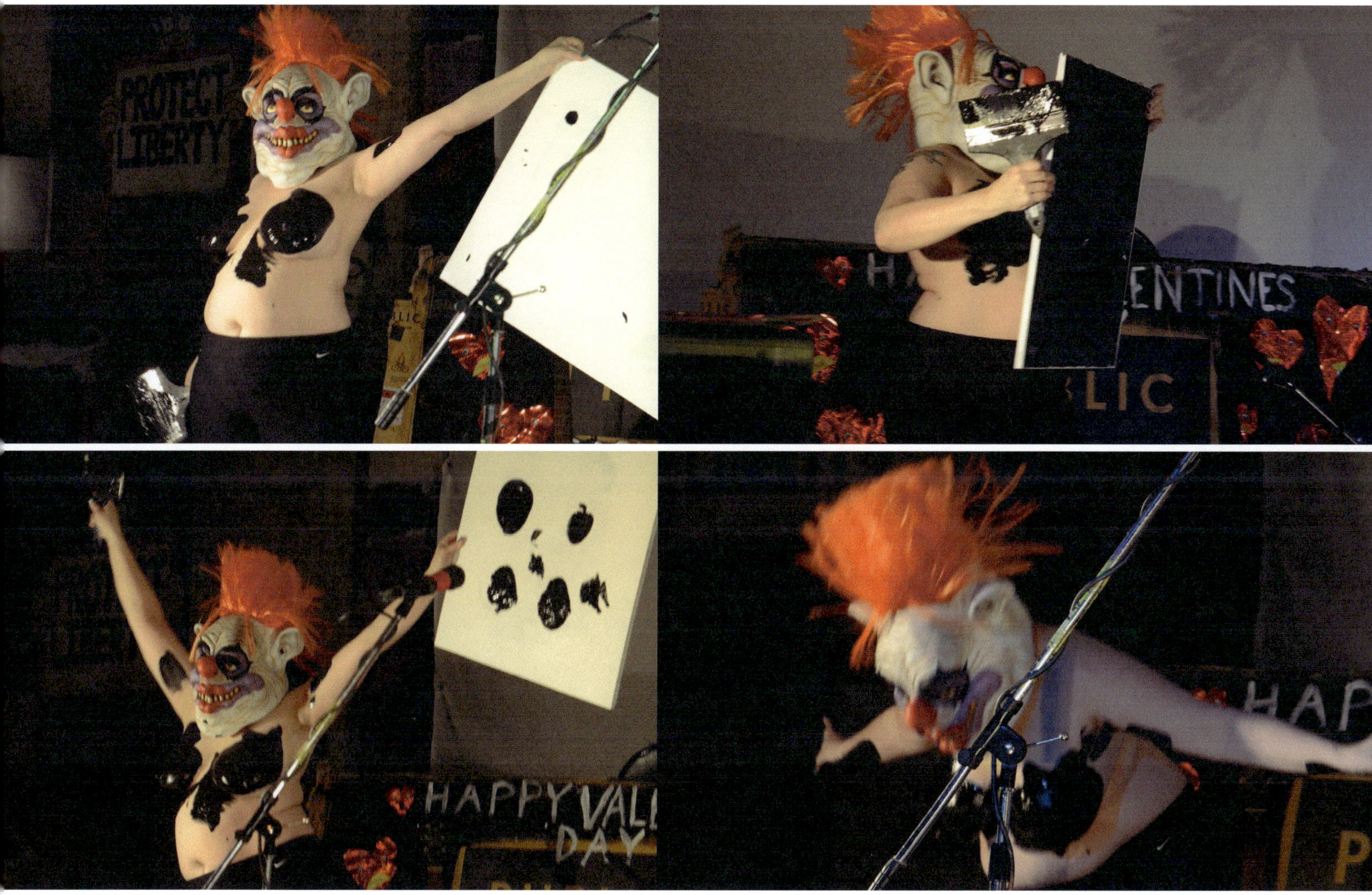

Cancer is Like...
Performance at Super Happy Fun Land, Houston, Texas
Feb 14, 2014
photos: Mitch Pengra

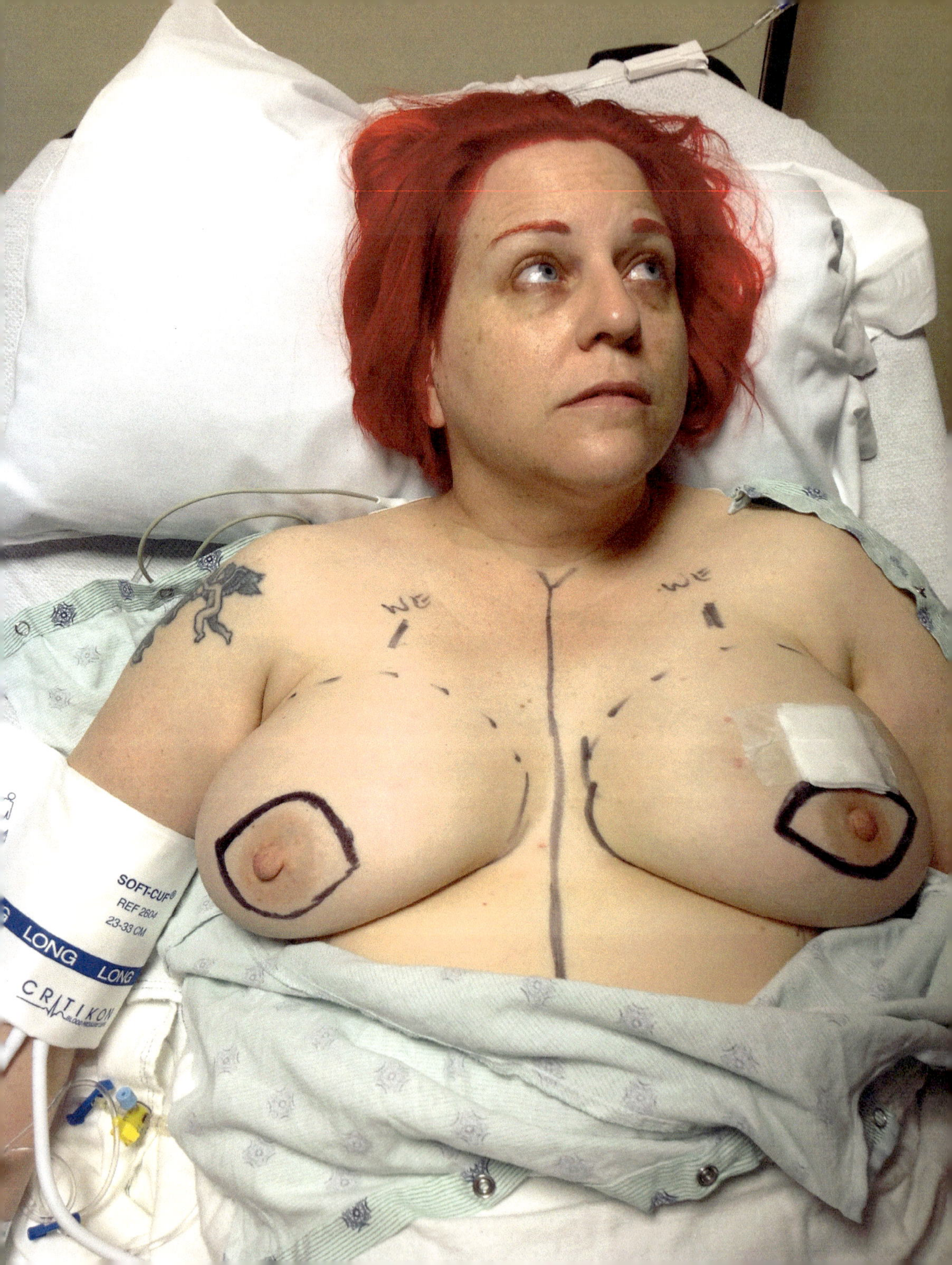
SOFT-CUF®
REF 2604
23-33 CM
LONG
LONG
CRITIKON

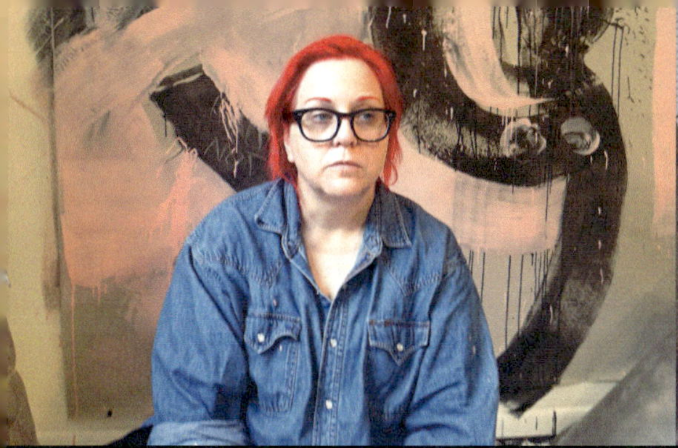

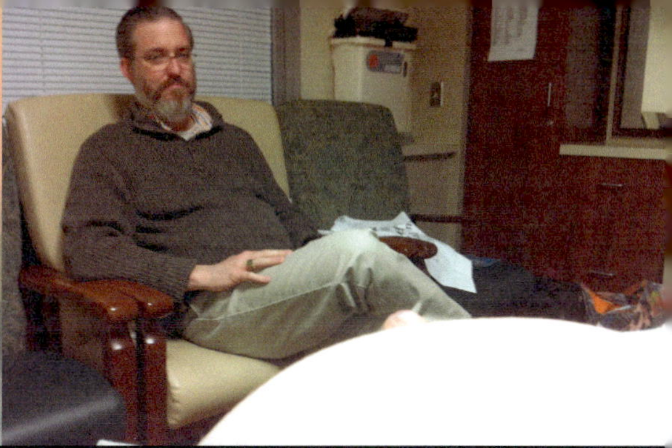

 love you Thedra! You are gonna do great tomorrow! I will be obsessively thinking about you al day. I'll be thinking about you tomorrow morning - yay us!!! Good luck Thedra!! (Monday morning already over here :-)) Love you! I will keep you and your surgeons in my prayers... I trust all wil go well. I love you and will be thinking about you every minute! I hope Stephen will call me the moment you're out of surgery. Big long loving hug, dear one! Love you Thedra Love you Thedra Lots of HUGS & LOVE to you, Thedra!!! Sending lots of love and positive thoughts to you! Thinking of you and sending pink healing light your way. Surrounding you in a bubble of love and positive energy, sister. Ill be thinking about you all day today. Xoxoxoxo so much love I love you, Thedra We are with you! Thinking of you today. Blessings Thinking of you today!!!!!!!!! My mama and I are making y'all dinner Wednesday and bringing it in for you all Thursday for your Thursday dinner Don't worry, she's supervising. Love you! Stay strong, lady. Our love and thoughts are with you dear! Love you lady!!! LOVE, LOVE, LOVE, LOVE! Couldn't sleep, finally got up early to sit and fret You are so precious to me and incredibly brave! Thinking of you, love and healing prayers. xxxooc sending love and healing energy your way Love you!! Good luck. Sending you positive vibes praying for you. I hope it all goes OK. Praying for Stephen too. Can't be easy on him either. We're thinking of you. Best of luck....thoughts are with you today... Lots of positive love your way Sending Positive Vibes and Healing Thoughts and Prayers to You. Asking The Great Archangel's Michae and Raphael to hang with you and surround you and your family with Comfort and Peace!!! Love & Light Awesome Lady!!! Thinking of you!! I am thinking you are at Methodist for your surgery all the Best Thadre I will be thinking of you and Praying for you . Love you Much love and positive energy being sent your way! xoxoxo You are on my mind and in my heart, thinking of you on this day, and sending prayers of love, peace and healing your way. Love you. thinking of the 2 of ya'll! love you XOXO This is not going to be fun, but you have a lot of love and support from a world of friends and family to help get you through. Hugs! xoxoxo Love and healing and strong thoughts sent you way Thedra... we are with you.... Praying praying praying You are in my prayers Thedra Cullar Ledford and your strength is a powerful thing to watch. Glitter energy on the way!xo Sending you love today. You go girl!!!! Looks like tons of love is flowing your way. We love you too! XXOO my beautiful friends Stephen and Thedra we send Love and keep your eye on the prize which is the bevy of brilliant dreams to come you have with your amazing family and your breathtaking art. Out Damn Spot! we Love you all. Sending you skinny warmth from cold NYC! xo Sending you healing prayers and all my love. We've got our feet planted firmly on the ground and our lip gloss on, and we're sending you all our love. Will be thinking of you all week. Sending super positive big get wel quick recovery vibes your way! Glad we connected all the best on new boobs Monday!

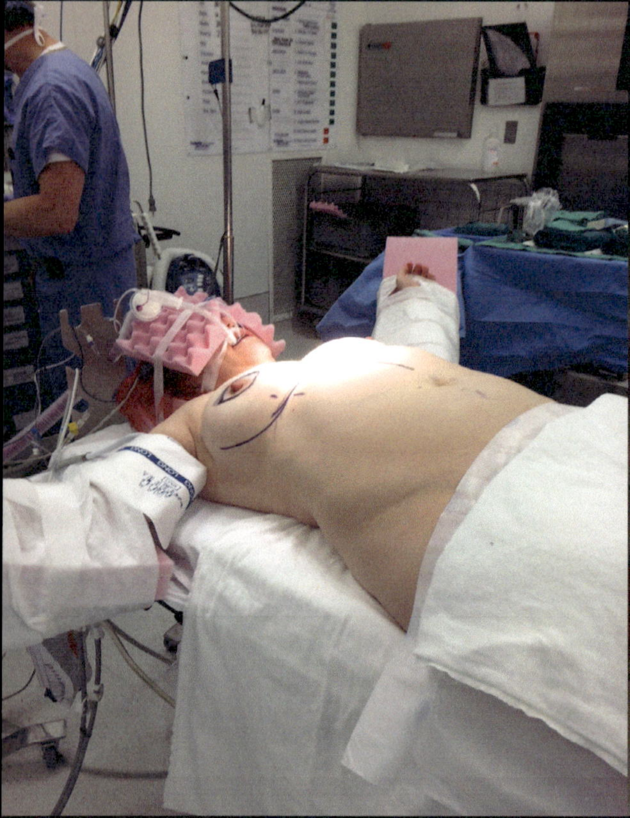

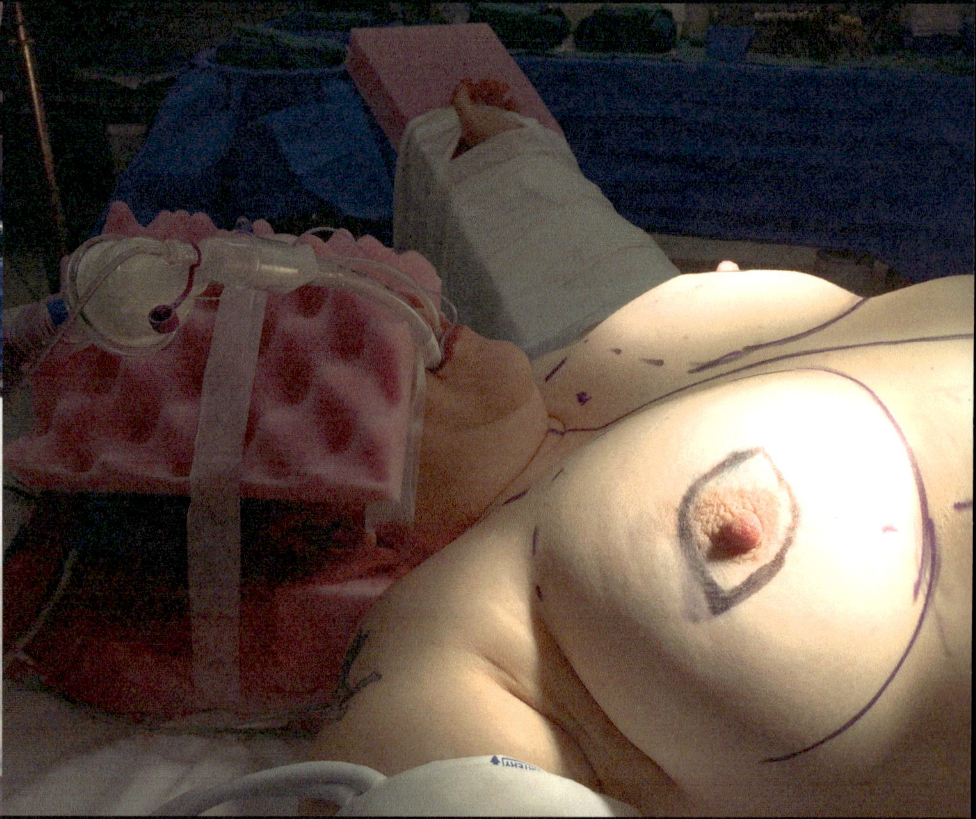

When you are about to go nuts and aggravated and in pain and sick if the poking and waking up and the trying to sleep and the noise and the light, remember we ALL Love you, and not that little sniveling kind of Love, we Love you with a BIG Love that is wonderful and abiding and mysterious and powerful. Because you are bigger than all this crap around you.... and this will pass. And Stephen is your brilliant knight who we Love equally. We are all out here pulling and crying and praying for you my darling. I promise, we are. I promise. from one cancer survivor to another. I promise.

Michelle Marie Engelman Berns

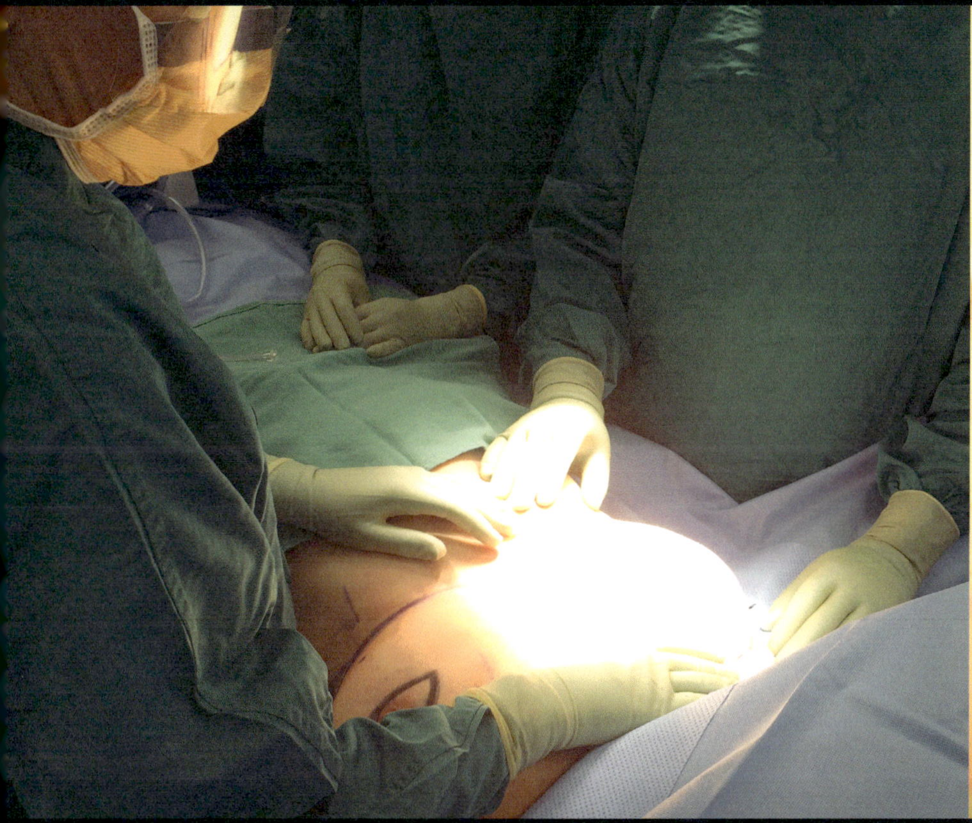

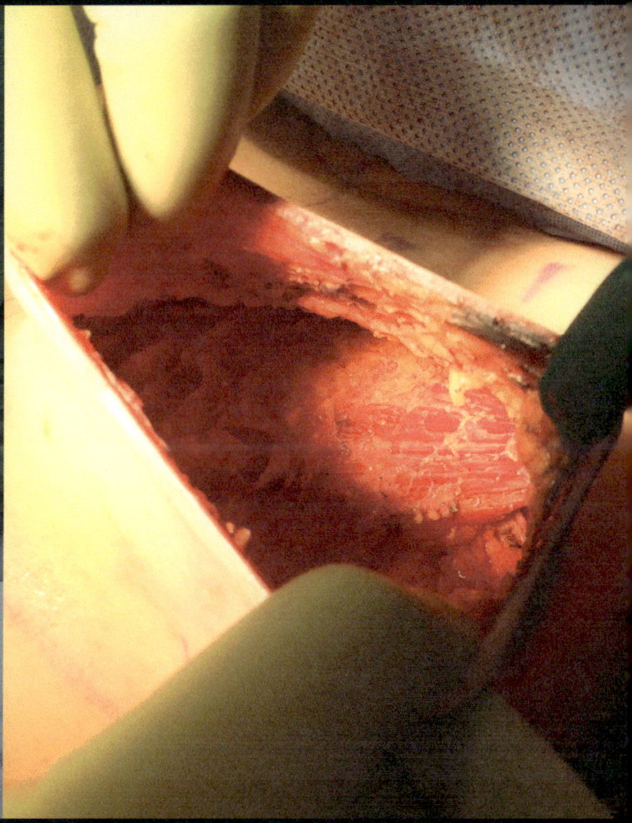

Bilateral Mastectomy
February 17, 2014
Photos: Dr. Barbara Bass

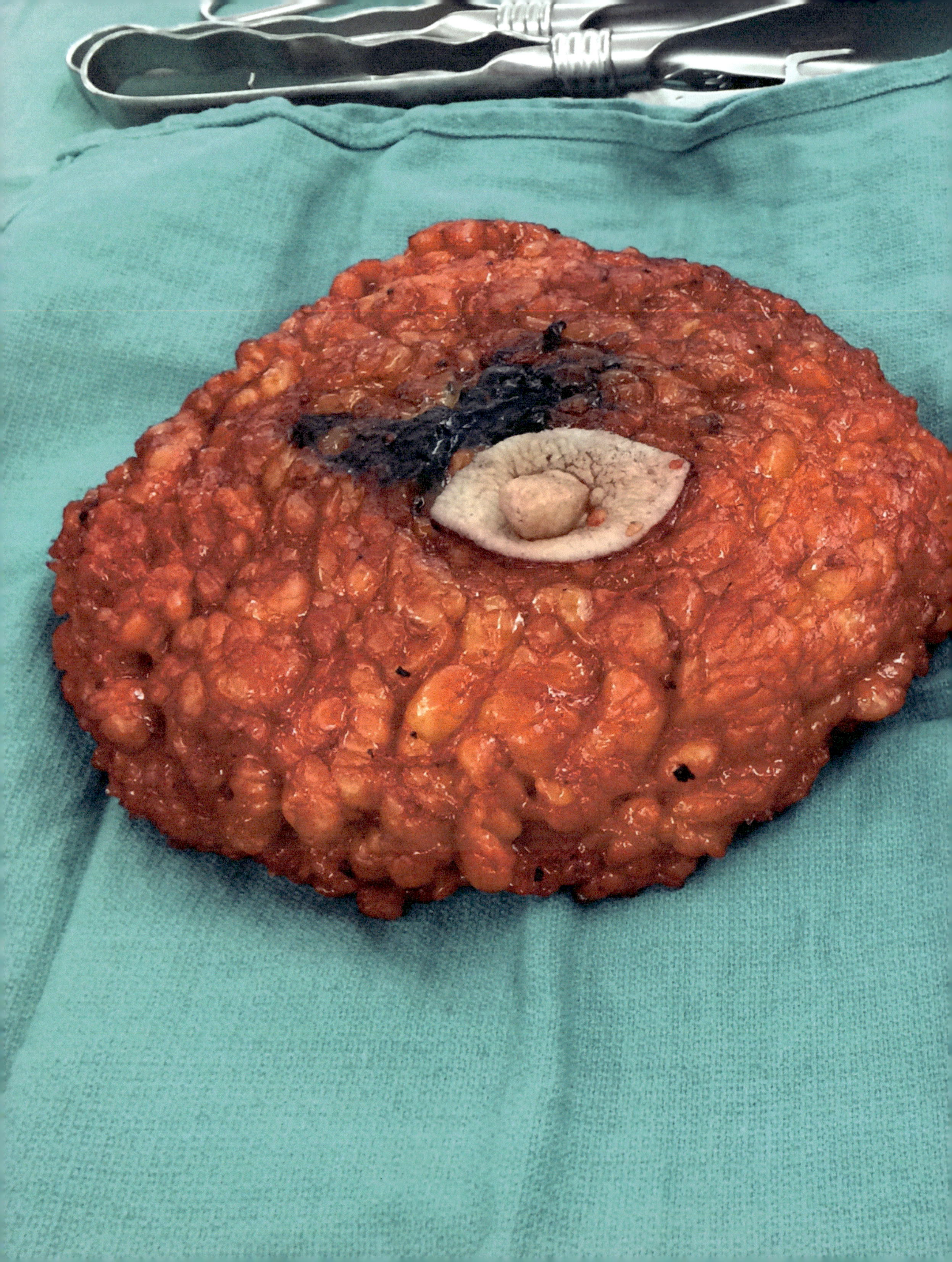

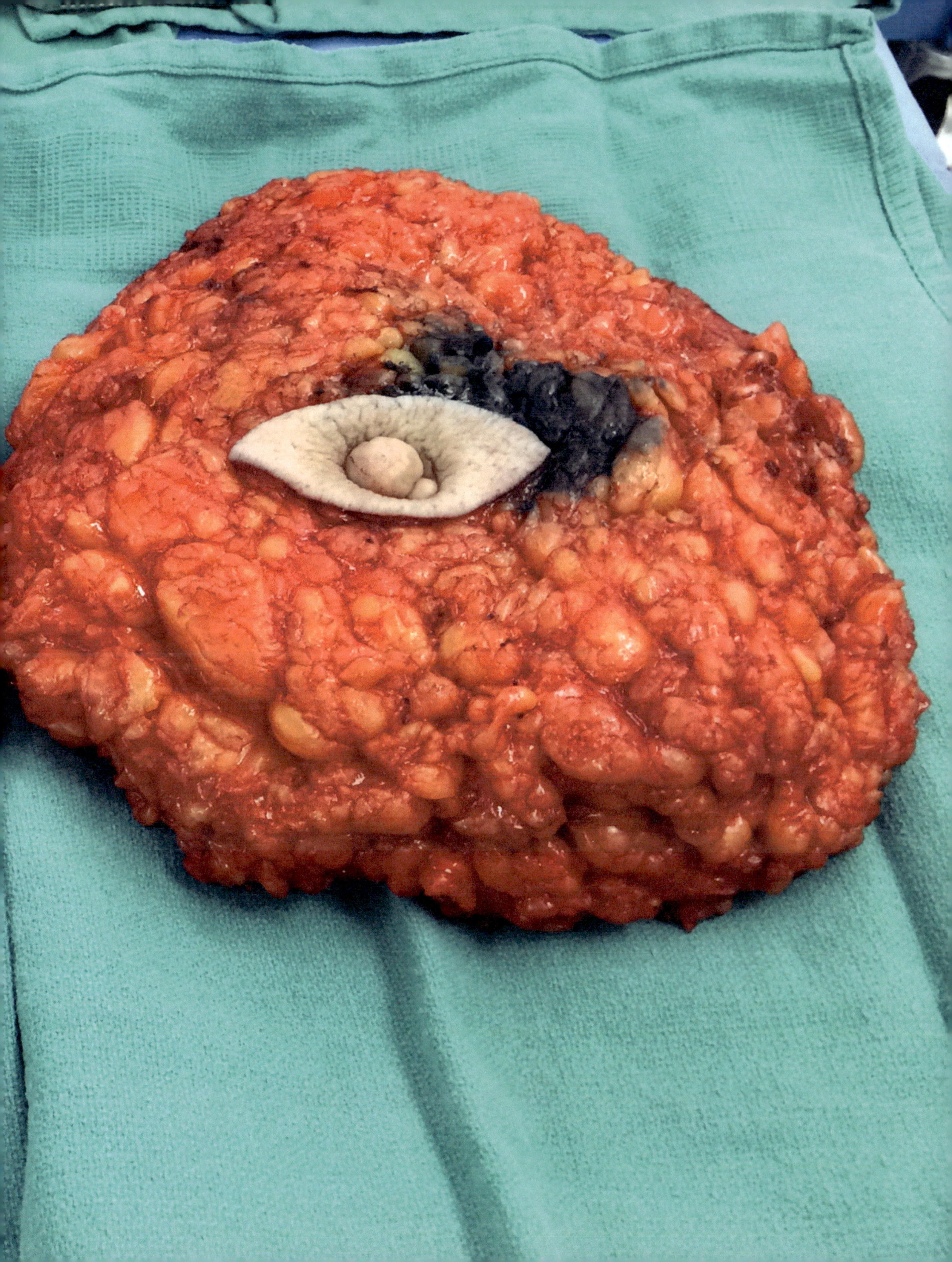

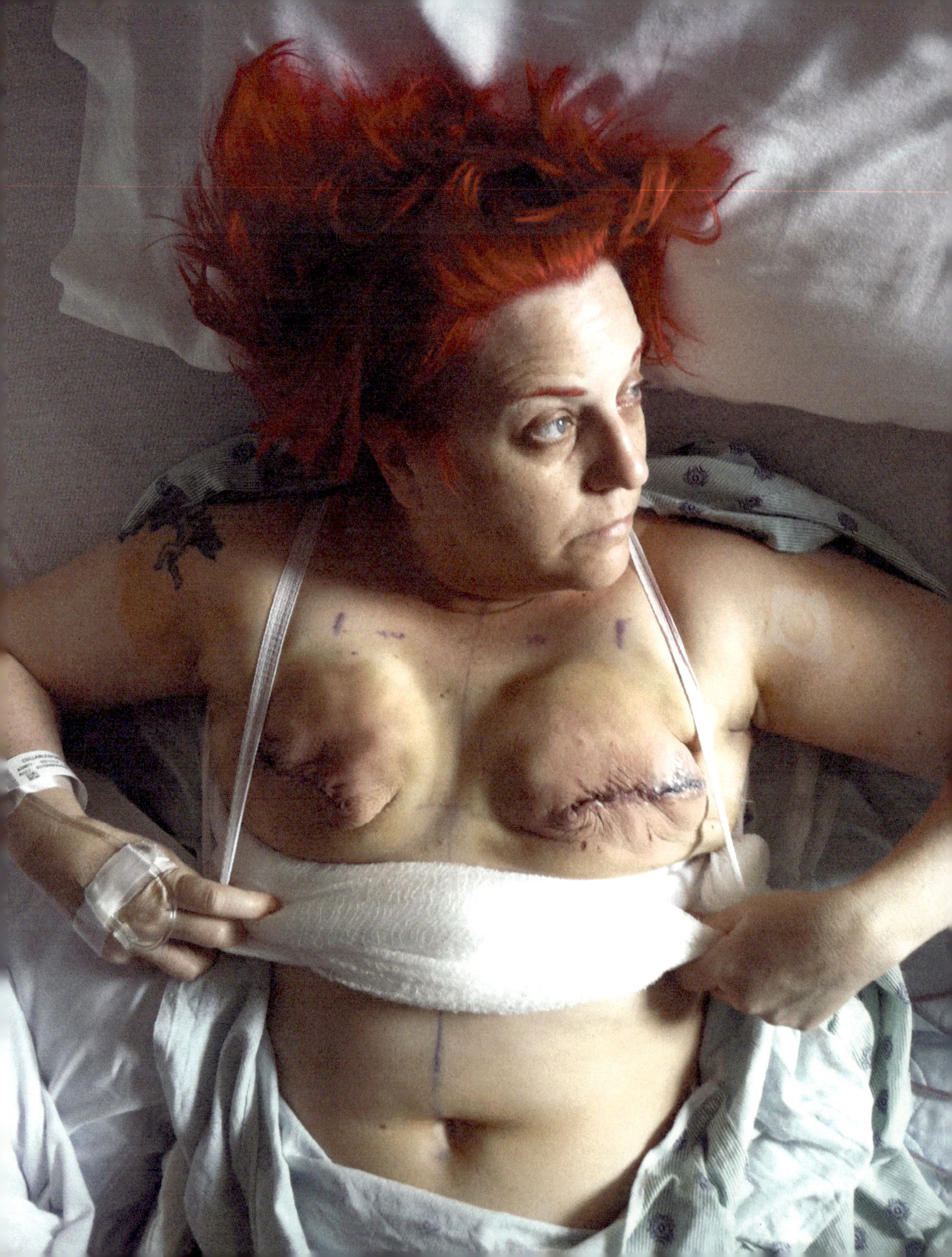

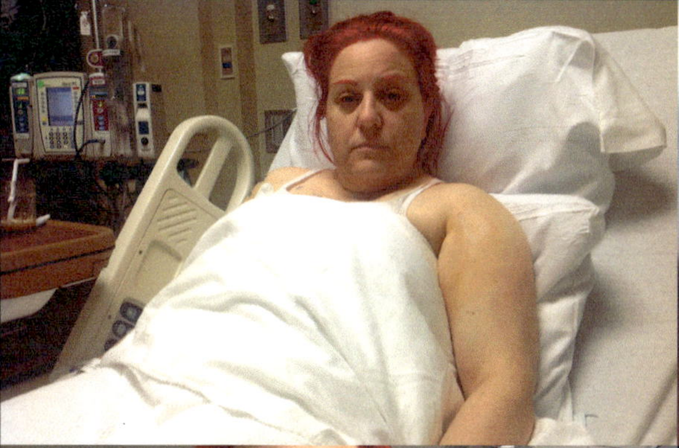
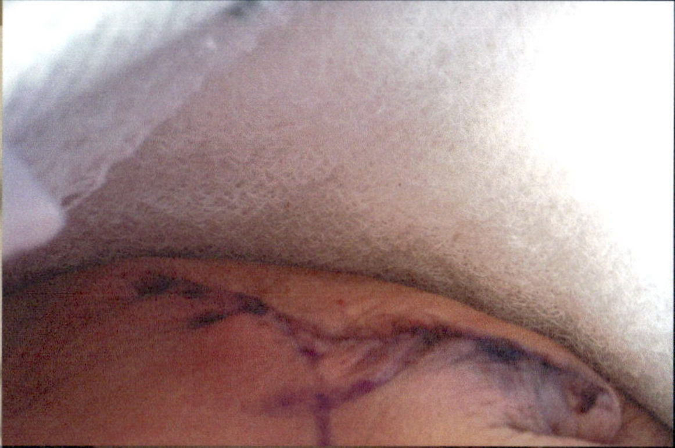
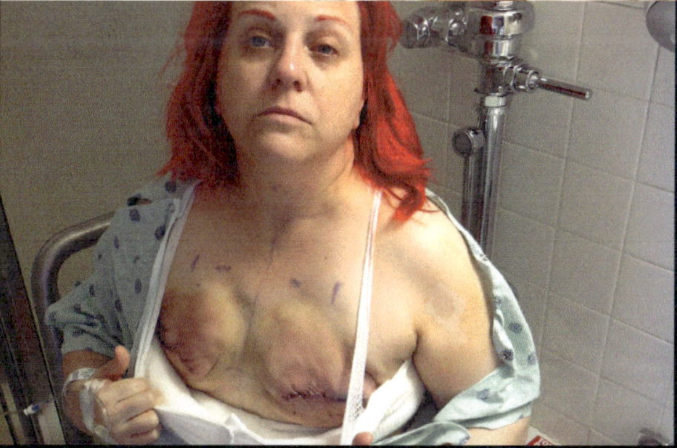
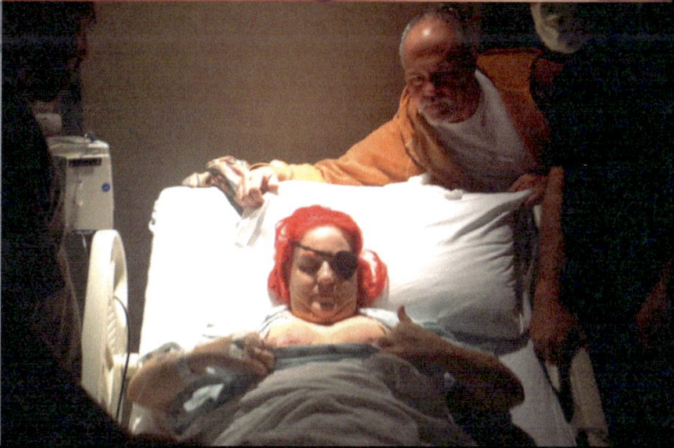

Removal operation complete, now starting reconstruction operation (two more hours.) All going well so far. No indication of cancer in lymph nodes, which is excellent news. Thanks to everyone for all the nice notes!

Thedra is now out of surgery and in recovery. The rest of her procedure was normal. All in all, the day has gone better than expected.

It took a long time to get released from the hospital, but Thedra is home now. She's uncomfortable and impatient, but that's to be expected. We're trying to get her 'nest' properly constructed and medicine routines figured out. She would love visitors, though she sleeps a lot. Again, thanks for all the well-wishes! We have the best friends anyone could hope to have.

Anatomic Pathology Diagnosis

The breast is serially sectioned from medial to lateral into 20 slices. The nipple is on slice 9. In slices 5-10, in the upper inner and upper outer quadrants, are five lesions, all of which have gross characteristics of invasive carcinoma.

Ink Code:
Blue - superficial margin, superior half of breast
Orange - superficial margin, inferior half of breast
Black - deep margin

There is a short suture designating superior, and a long suture designating lateral.

A. Lymph nodes, right axillary, sentinel node, excision

1. Benign lymph nodes (0/2)

B. Breast, right, prophylactic mastectomy

1. Ductal carcinoma in situ (DCIS)
   a. Multifocal in upper inner quadrant, lower inner quadrant, and midline at junction of lower inner and outer quadrants. Present focally in slices 14-22 of 23 slices. DCIS spans 8cm (greatly overestimates the volume of DCIS.)
   b. Cribriform and focal solid architectural patterns.
   c. Nuclear grades 1 and 2 (variable) of 3 by SBR criteria.
   d. Absent central comedo necrosis.
   e. Surgical margins free of carcinoma. Closest margins of DCIS: focally 5 mm from superficial and deep margins
2. Lobular carcinoma in situ (LCIS)
   a. 5 mm focus, upper outer quadrant
3. Atypical ductal hyperplasia (ADH)
   a. Cribriform architectural pattern. Focally associated with DCIS.
4. Atypical lobular hyperplasia (ALH)
   a. Pagetoid involvement of extralobular duct in nipple. Involvement of lobules, upper outer and inner quadrants.
5. Lobular neoplasia (ALH/LCIS)
   a. Present focally in 4 of 44 slides
6. Macrocysts and microcysts, multiple with associated apocrine metaplasia, including papillary apocrine metaplasia.
7. Columnar cell change. Lactational-like change, microfocal
8. Milium of nipple, 0.6 mm. No Paget's disease of the nipple seen. Microcalcifications, few, minute, calcium phosphate type, associated with benign lobules.

C. Lymph node, left axillary, sentinel, excision

1. Benign lymph nodes (0/2)

D. Breast, left, mastectomy

1. Invasive ductal carcinoma.
   a. 7 tumors. Multifocal, in slices 4-12 of 20 (mainly upper inner, upper central and medial third of upper outer quadrant.) Multifocal, spanning 8 cm, noncontiguous foci.
   b. 1.95 cm carcinoma, in upper inner and outer quadrants, associate with biopsy clip (designated first lesion)
   c. 1.5 cm carcinoma, upper inner quadrant (designated second lesion) 1.4 cm carcinoma, upper central (designated third lesion.)
   d. 1.9 cm carcinoma, in upper inner and outer quadrants, associated with biopsy clip (designated fourth lesion)
   e. 1.7 cm carcinoma, upper central to upper outer quadrant (designated fifth lesion)
   f. 1.0 cm carcinoma, lower outer quadrant (designated sixth lesion)
   g. 1.2 cm carcinoma, upper outer quadrant (designated seventh lesion)
   h. Elston-Ellis modified SBR score 3+2+1 = 6 of 9
   i. Histologic grade 2 of 3
   j. Mitotic index = 0.3 (average mitoses per high power field)
2. Surgical margins free of carcinoma
   a. Closest margins: invasive carcinoma and DCIS 3.5 mm from superficial margin, upper inner quadrant. Pleomorphic LCIS focally 3 mm from superficial margin, upper outer quadrant

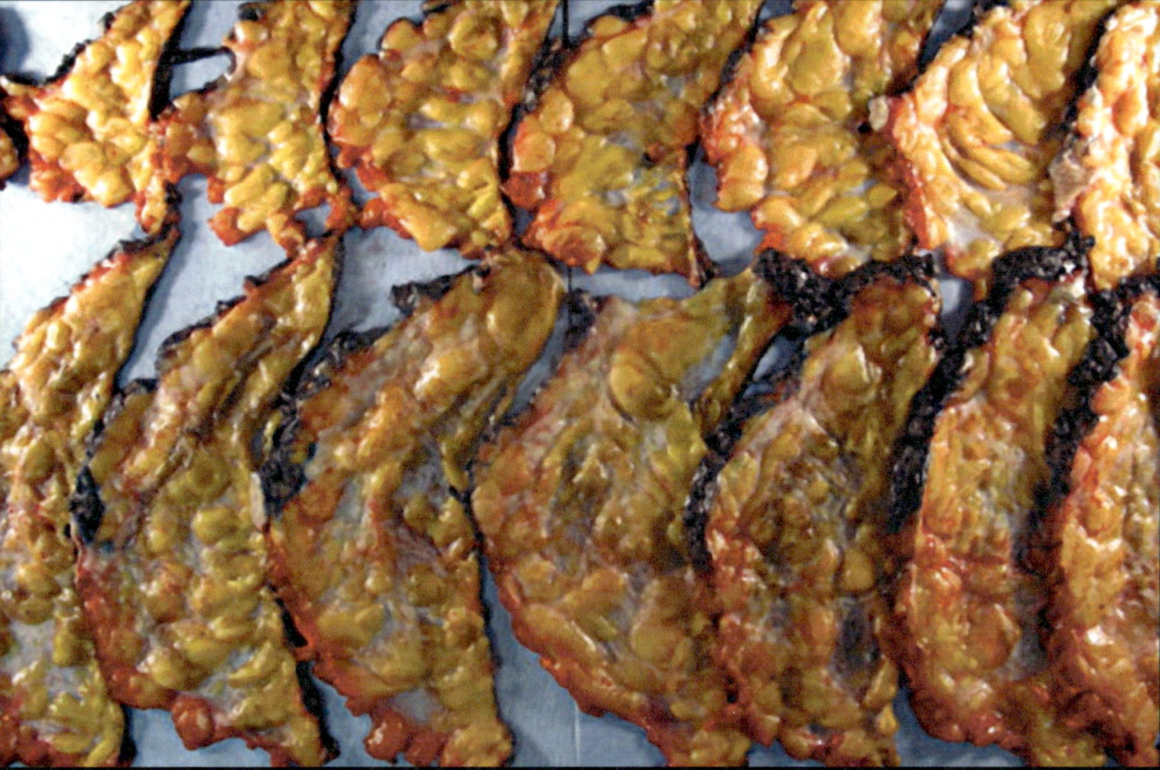

The white bits are calcifications from cancer, not reflections. I'm never eating bacon again.

Pathologist's Report
(Whitman's Sampler)
Dr. Mary Schwartz
This was all completely over my head. I was either swiveling around on the doctor's stool or in the gift shop during these discussions. Thank God Stephen was taking good notes. (Did I

February 26, 2014

Had two appointments yesterday, first with the plastic surgeon (yawn), then with the primary surgeon (wow!)

You may remember that I decided to have both boobs chopped off to stay symmetrical, even though only the left one was a troublemaker. It turns out that the right one was not nearly as innocent as it had been pretending to be. It had been harboring DCIS, some LCIS, a little ADH, and a dash of ALH/LCIS. All of these are different forms of cancers, though none of them are invasive. It was a Whitman's Sampler box, "totally* full" of cancers that surprised all of my doctors.

As for the left one, they didn't find three tumors they expected, but they found seven (!) ranging from 1 cm to 1.95 cm in size. They also found quite a bit of DCIS, but we knew that was coming.

While all of this could have been very bad news, there are three very important, and very good things that made yesterday a great day. First, I had both boobs removed (I'm the kind of girl who like matching bedside tables.) Second, none of the lymph nodes on either side have any cancer in them at all. Since the lymph nodes are how cancer spreads throughout the body, this means that it has not spread. Finally, no cancer was found around "the margins" of the surgery area. In other words, it appears that they got all of it.

The big question to be answered now is whether or not chemo will be needed, and there is not an obvious answer at this point. They are going to do more analysis of all the tumors, and genetic testing of several of them to find out if they are all of a similar, well-behaved and unaggressive type. If so, then chemo is unlikely. If, however, there is even one of the little fuckers that is aggressive, the decision becomes trickier. We'll know more in a couple of weeks.

Tumor Board Discussion

The focus of the debate had to do with how to "stage" my cancer. There are two ways of doing that assessment: by the size of the largest tumor (1.9 cm) or, by the total size of ALL the tumors (over 6 cm.) If they use the first approach, I have "stage one" cancer that would not require chemotherapy. If they use the second approach, I have "stage two" cancer that does require chemotherapy.

The winning argument seems to be that a large tumor behaves very differently from a small tumor. It is large because it is more aggressive. Small tumors, especially my slow-growing kind, aren't doing that. They have therefore staged my cancer at stage one, but they are submitting samples of my largest tumors for a complete genetic workup. The expectation is that all of the tumors are of the same type, but the genetic test will determine that.

In other words, once I have this next surgery, I'm done with my cancer odyssey. I will have to take Tomoxafin for the next ten years to block progesterone and estrogen (which was feeding my cancers), but the primary side-effects of that drug shouldn't effect me too badly.

Believe it or not, yesterday was a freaky and fantastic day, full of crazy and wonderful chance encounters and meaningful conversations.

Thanks to all of you!

(* actual word the doctor used.)

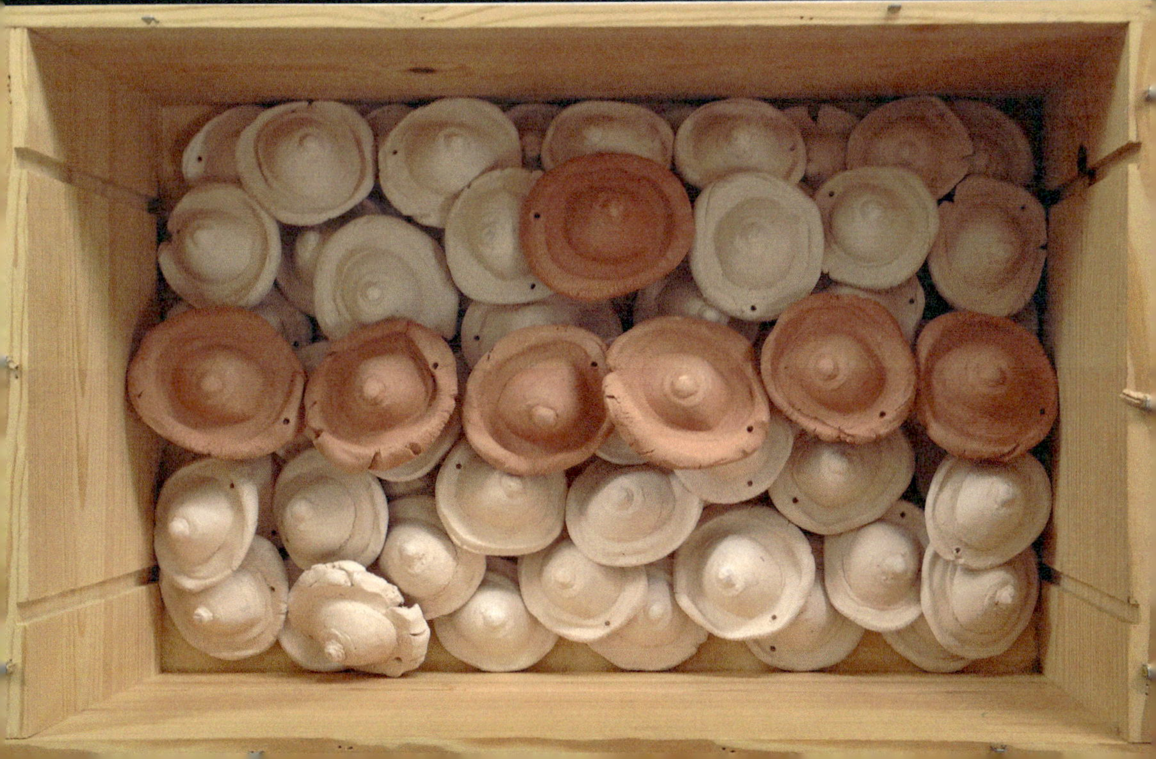

If my plastic surgeon had spent ten more minutes getting to know me I would have never gone with reconstruction. He kept arguing with me and saying "you'll be concave." I kept saying that I just wanted to be flat. Since this was all being provided for free, I felt compelled to be quiet, and to go along with what he wanted to do. I finally said "OK, just an 'A.'"

In the week and a half after surgery, I learned that there would be no nipple, there would be no feeling, that it can take six or even nine procedures to finish reconstruction, that implants can hide new tumors, and that you have to replace them every 10 years.

Why, when they just removed cancer from your body, would you want to have some PLASTIC put right back in there? Hmmm, what's a common carcinogen?... PLASTIC?

I equate it to this: My son has died, lets stuff him and prop him up in the corner so that nobody else notices that he's gone. Why all this trouble so that society can be happy thinking that nothing had ever gone wrong?

I knew going in to my follow-up appointment with my plastic surgeon that he was not going to like what I was planning to tell him, so I recorded it. We've only been able to listen to this once because it upsets my husband and I so much.

I now know that my experience was not uncommon. Dealing with how fucked up that is will be a whole other body of work.

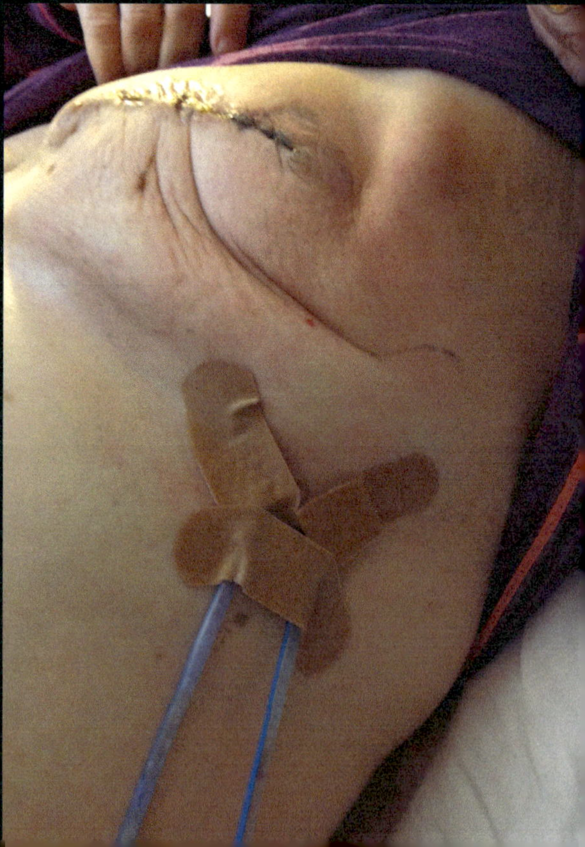

March 10, 2014

About three weeks post surgery, I started to develop an infection in the left one that was causing not only pain, but weakness and dizziness. On Friday, the plastics doctor asked me to go into the ER at Methodist, not because I had an emergency but because that was the easiest way for them to get a good look at me.

The ER doctor still had to check me out. He pretty much only wanted to make sure I wasn't dying right then, but then we started talking. He enjoyed the whole kidney/finding cancer story, but wasn't all that surprised. He said that in the normal course of treating emergency cases he finds cancer two or three times a month that the patients didn't know they had.

Miscommunication among the ER, my surgeon, and the plastics doctor meant that my surgeon, Dr. Bass, was the first one to show up. I think she was concerned that the drains were causing more harm than good. Though the drains were still removing fluids that needed to come out, the plastic tubes also offered a pathway for infection. She decided to remove the drains, even though the plastics doctor was the one responsible for them. I felt better.

When the plastics resident finally arrived at the ER (he had been sitting around waiting for the call for hours) he seemed to have concerns about the drains being removed. A few hours afterwards, we got a call from the plastics doctor's nurse telling us to be very, very vigilant over the weeked about potential problems. We should immediately go to the ER if we saw any of these symptoms. She scheduled an appointment early Monday morning.

Over the weekend, we did notice these symptoms and called in to find out whether an ER visit was necessary. The on-call doctor said to stay at home both times.

Monday morning, as instructed, I drove out to Katy to have my appointment with the plastic surgeon. They were concerned about infection, and I was not feeling well. After examining me, he decided to do the second surgery, to remove the expanders, the next morning.

We got all our paperwork and were headed out to the car when I basically collapsed. I couldn't make it to the car, let alone to home overnight. A kind nurse who was walking by noticed and escorted me to the emergency room and got some fluids into me. She arranged to have me admitted immediately.

The room was four star! Corner suite with nice windows and a seperate room for Stephen to sleep in. (He really needed it — we had stayed up all night watching for infection and nursing me through.)

In the morning, I had the surgery which went very smoothly. The painkillers worked well and the recovery was much easier. I was up wandering around the next day. I immediately felt like the toxic shit had been removed.

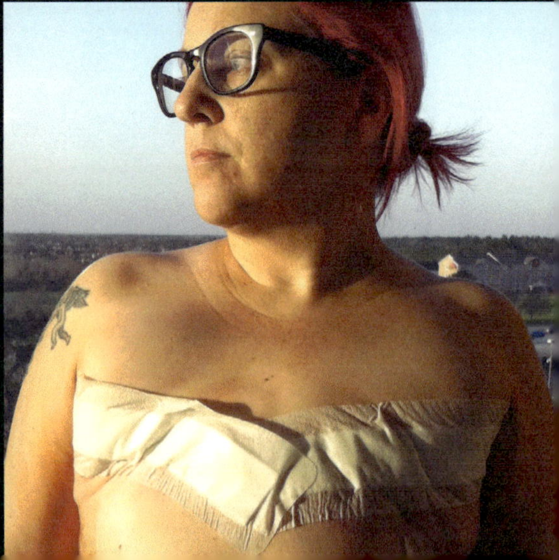

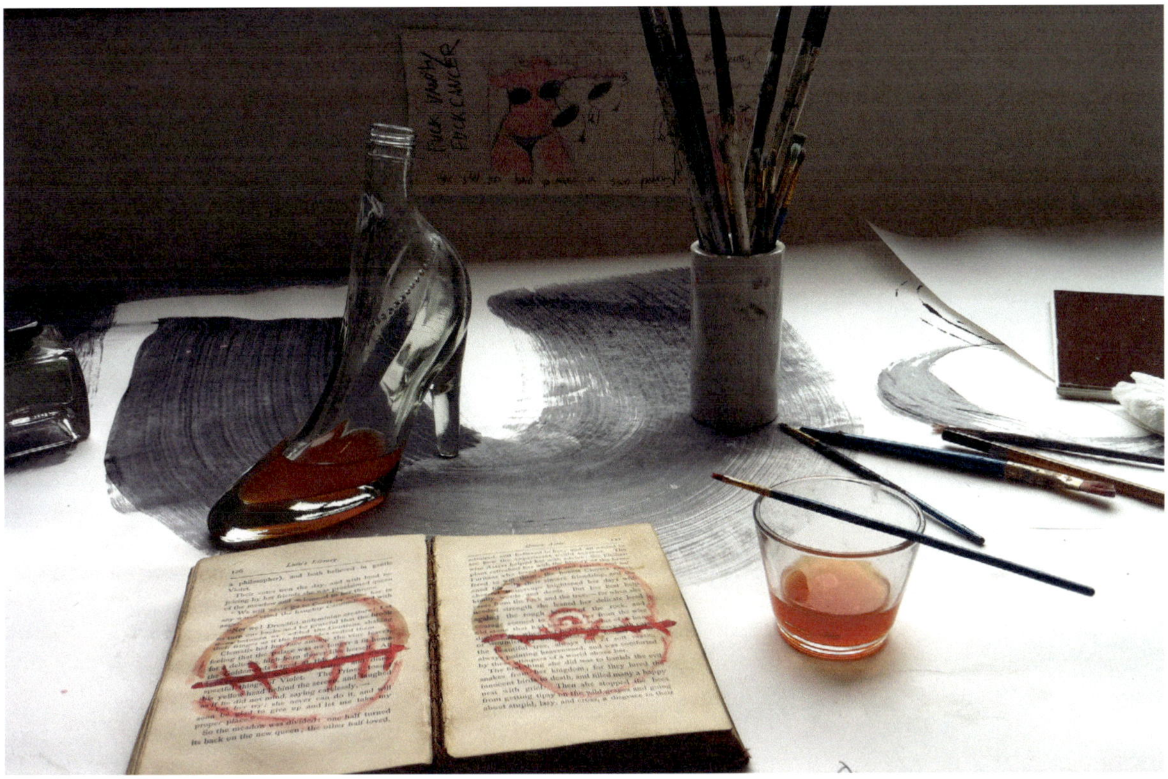

De-Juicing Book
2014, 6"x9"x 2"
Old book, bodily fluid

In the three weeks following surgery, Stephen had to strip the lines, empty my surgical drains, and note the volumes. This twice-daily process was always very emotional for me, so I would take a Xanax and continue with our binge-watching *Downton Abbey*. I started collecting these "juices" and ended up doing a few pieces with it as ink.

Dolls
2014
Mixed media
It feels like I am turning into one of my old dolls

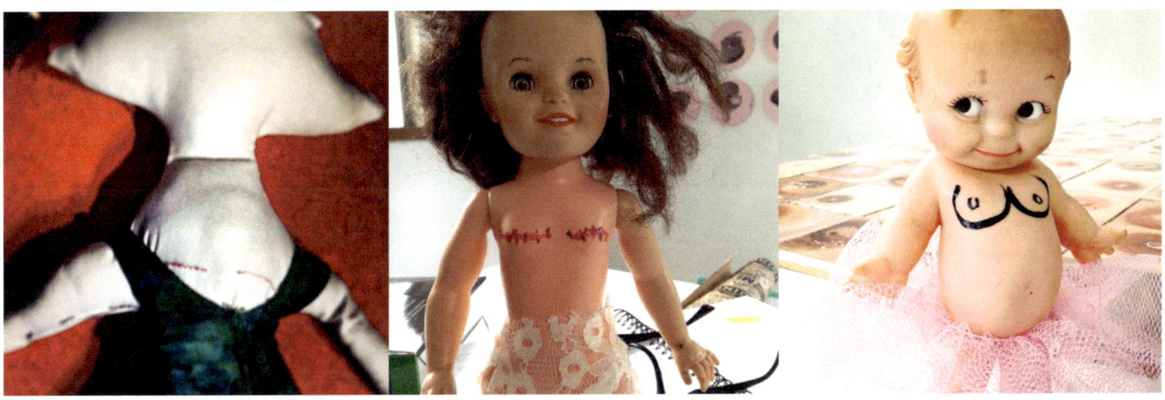

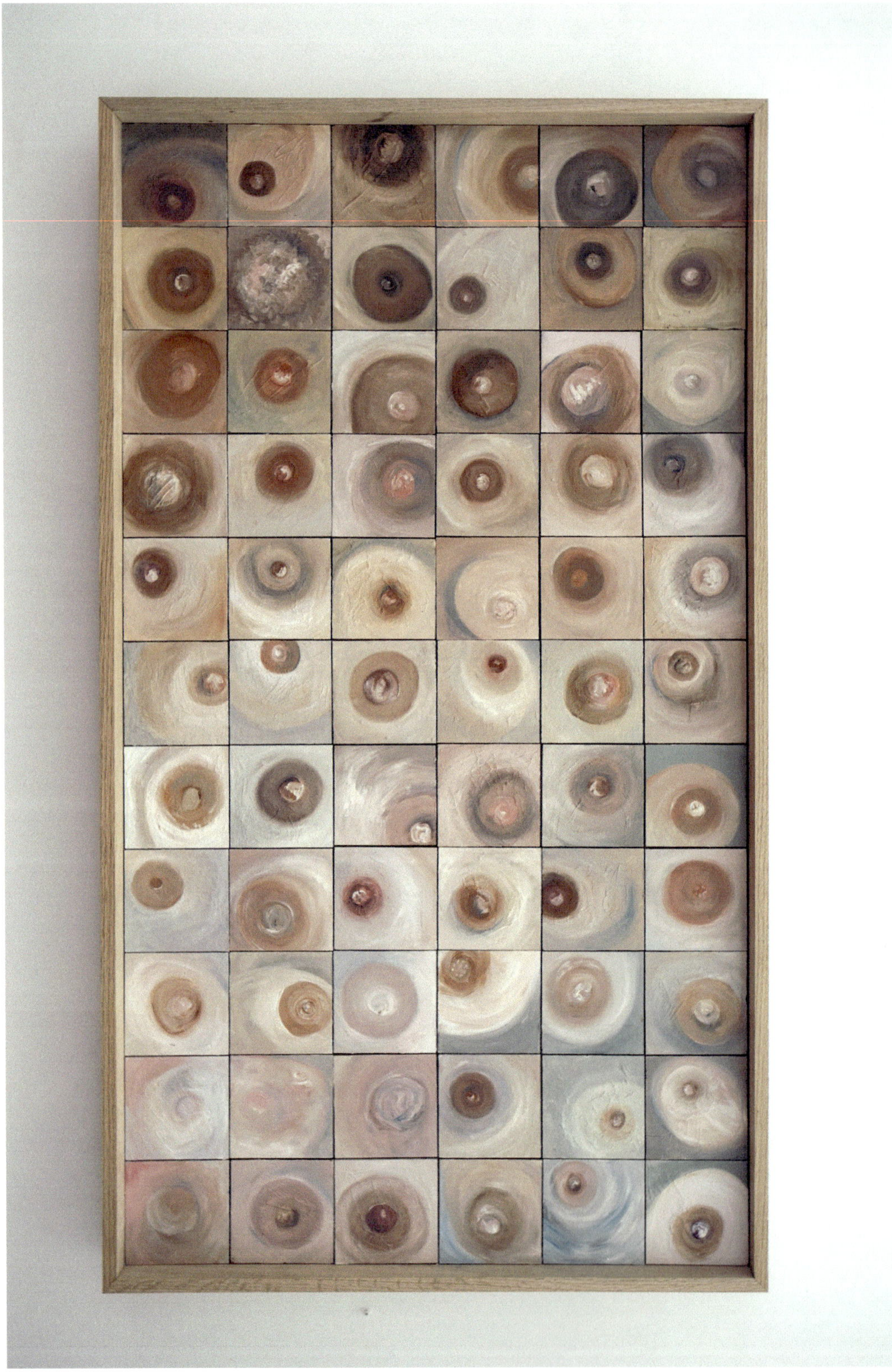

Front Nipples
2014, 34" x 62"
Oil on wood

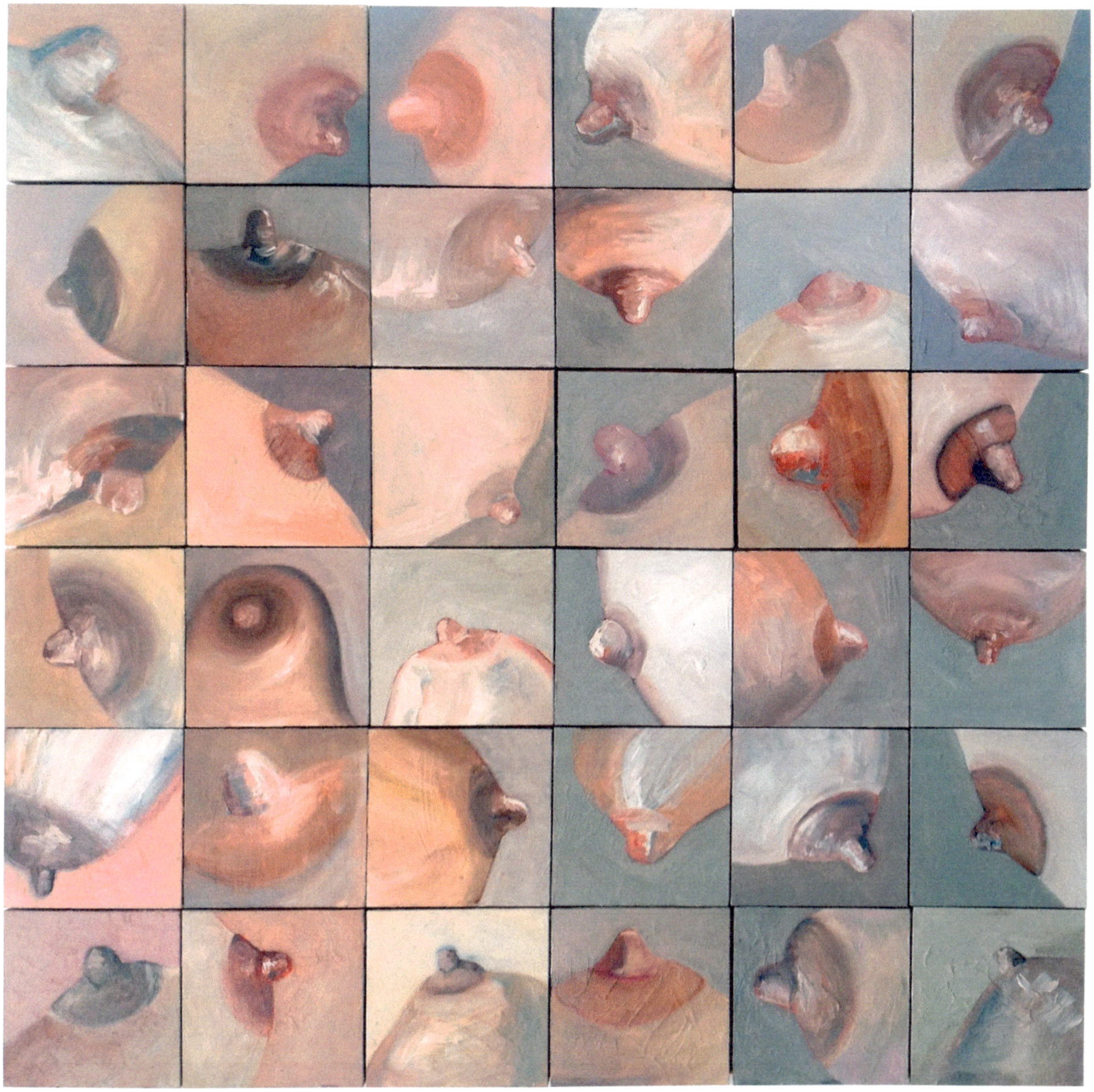

Side Nipples
Oil on wood
2014, 34" x 34"
These were mostly therapy and a distraction for me after my surgery. I could sit in one place and paint them for hours without exerting myself very much. Over time, they accumulated and became a mosaic. Since my surgery I have become as obsessed with breasts as a teenage boy.

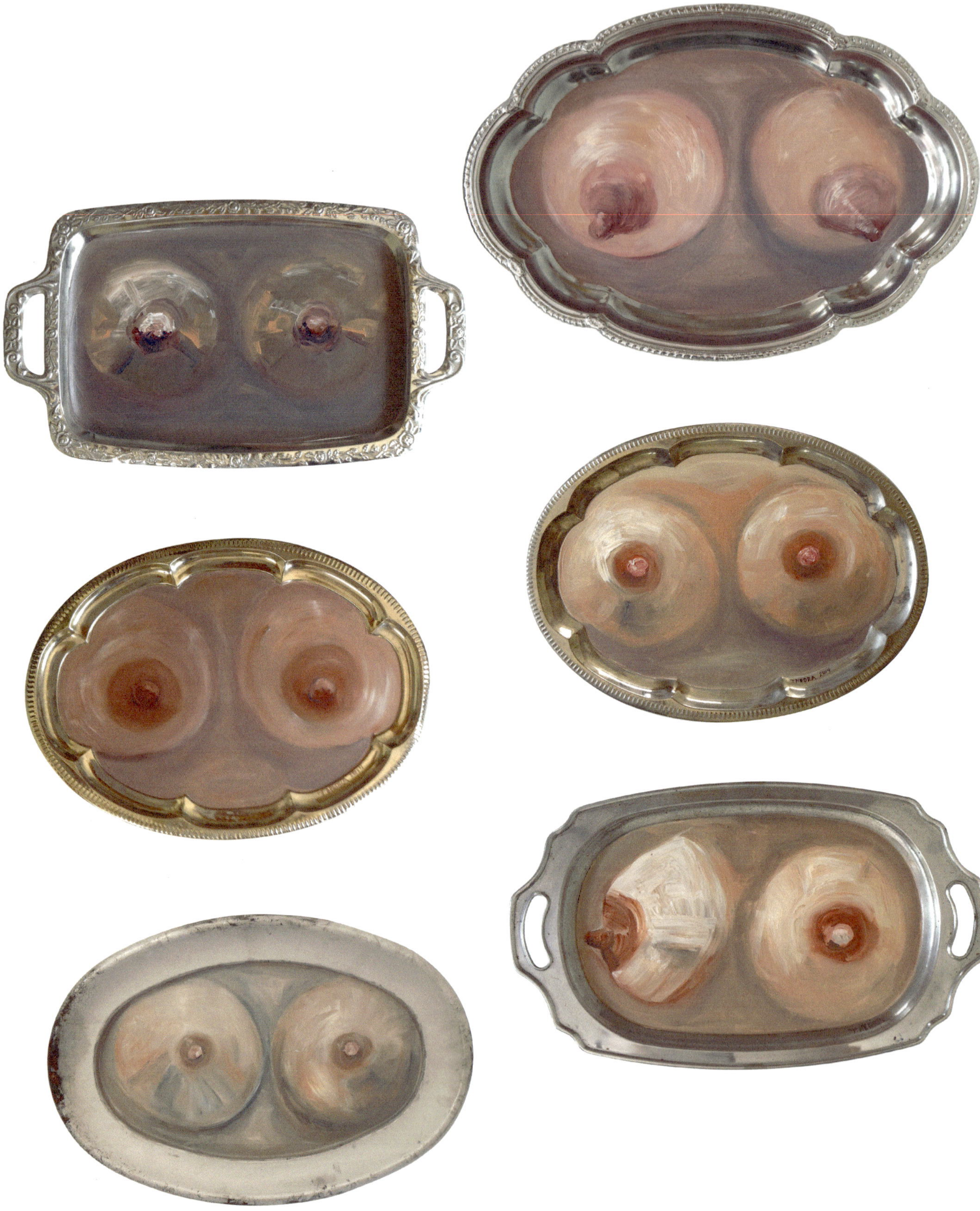

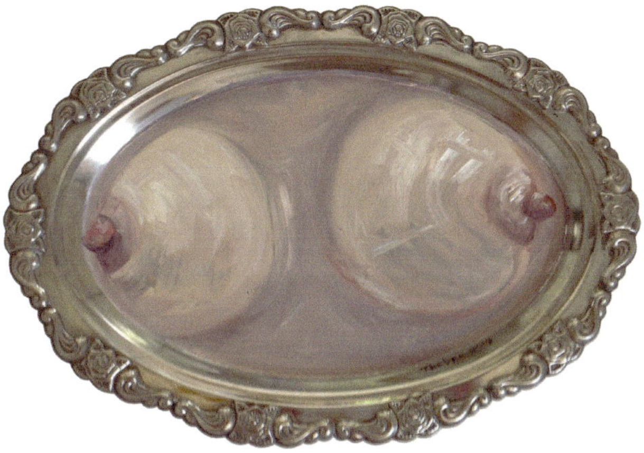
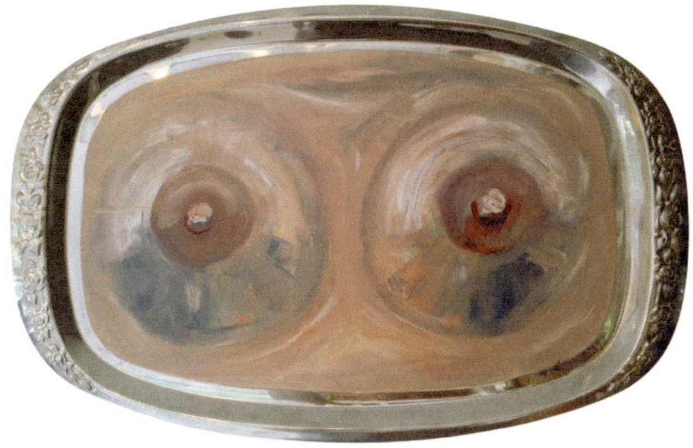
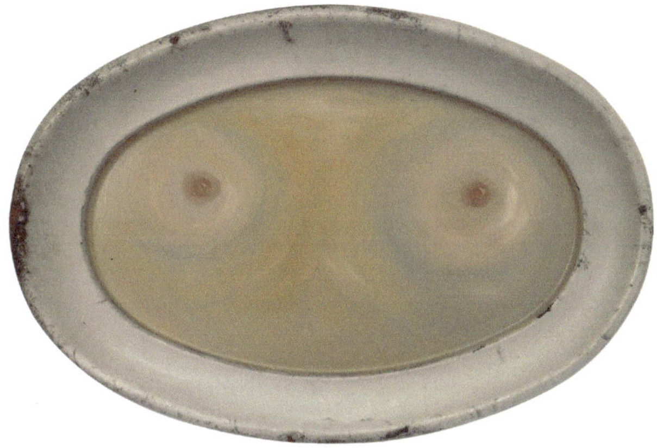
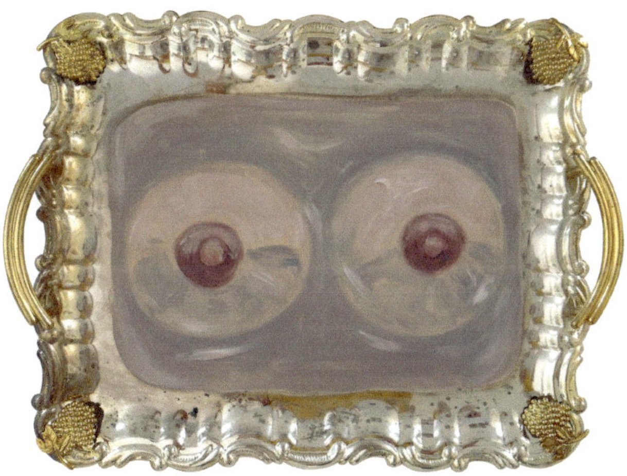
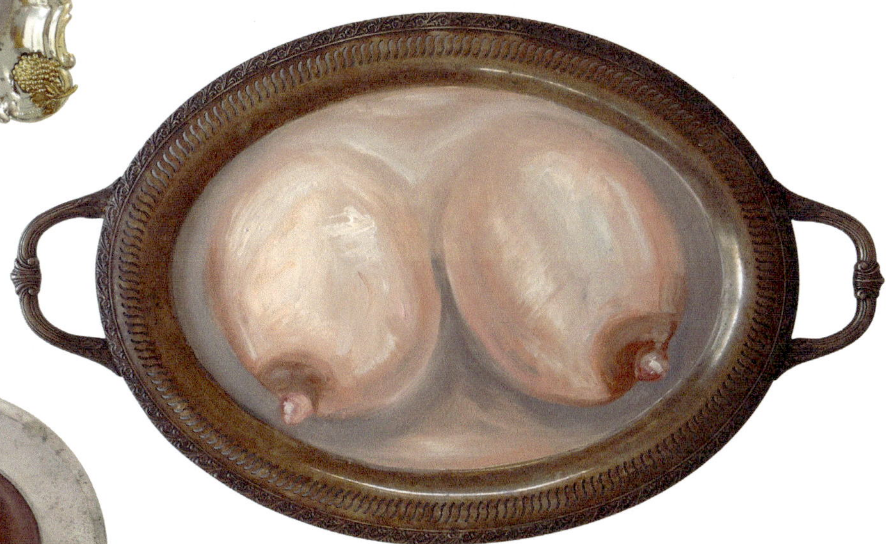
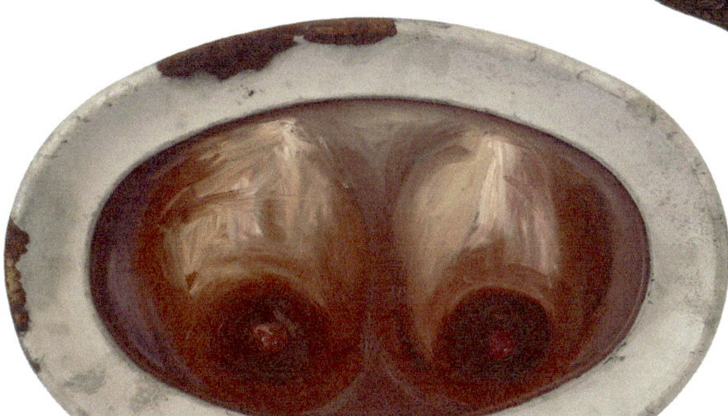

Platters
2014-2015, sizes vary
Oil on metal serving trays
My ongoing tribute to St. Agatha. So far, there are 36 completed.

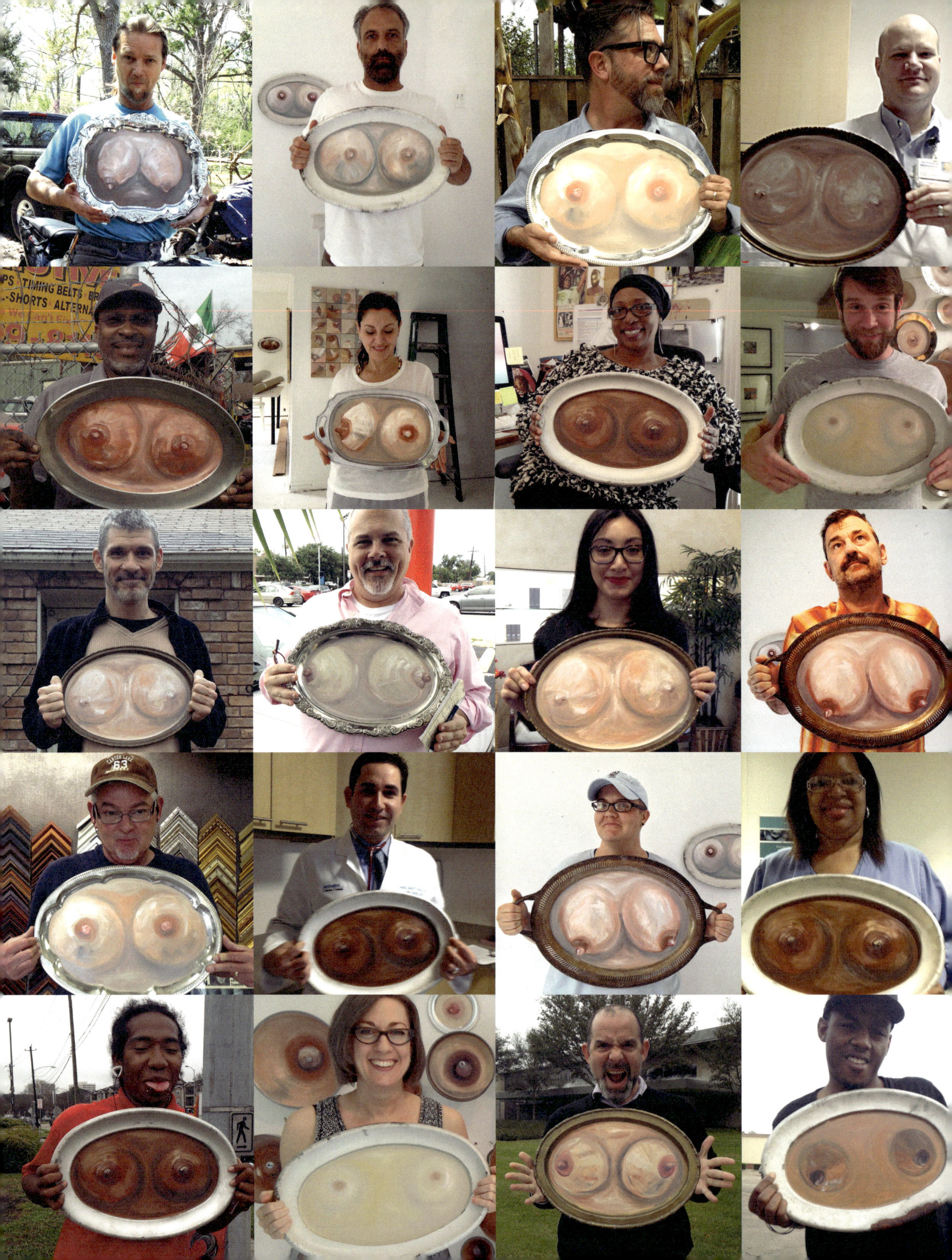
TIMING BELTS
63

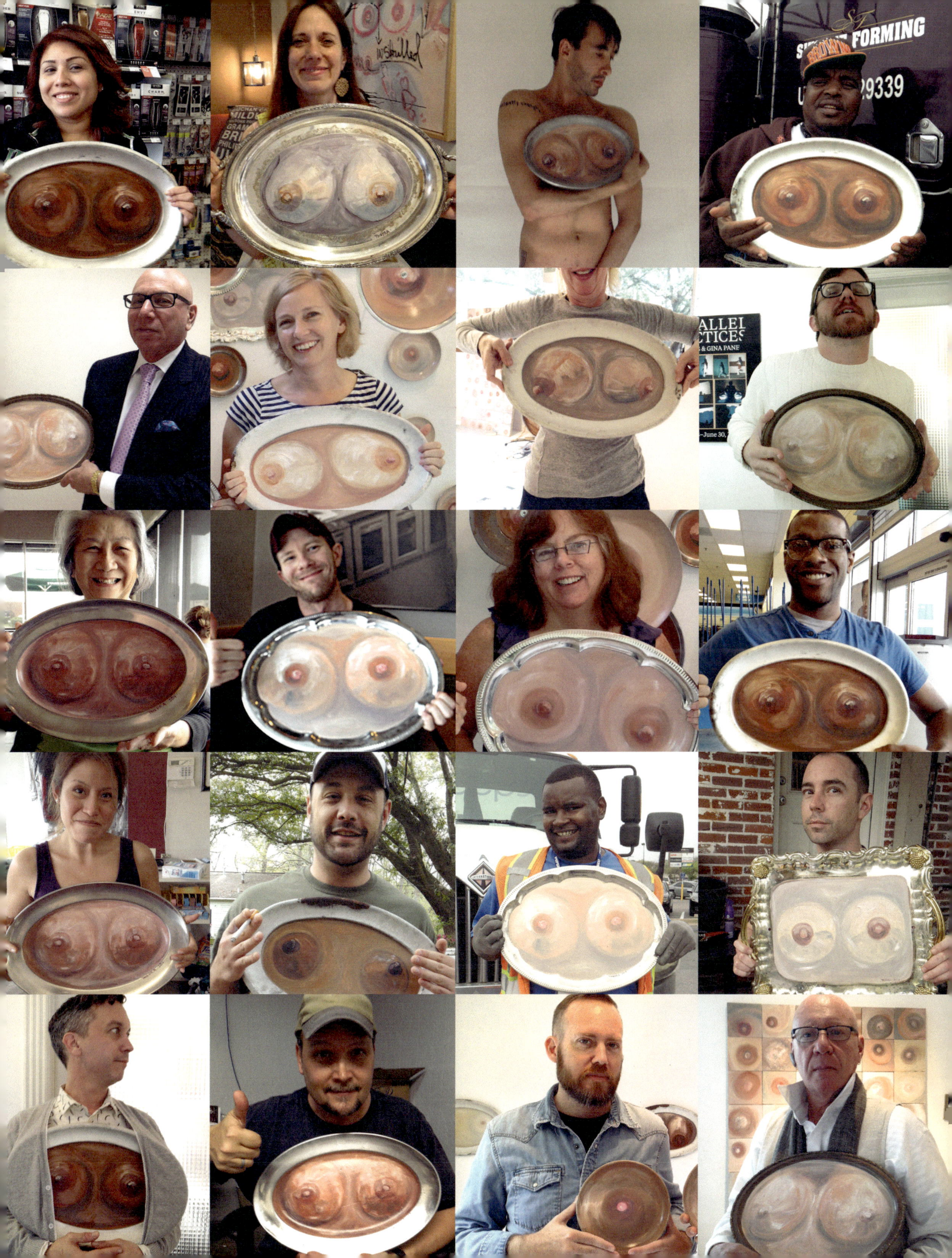
FORMING
& GINA PANE

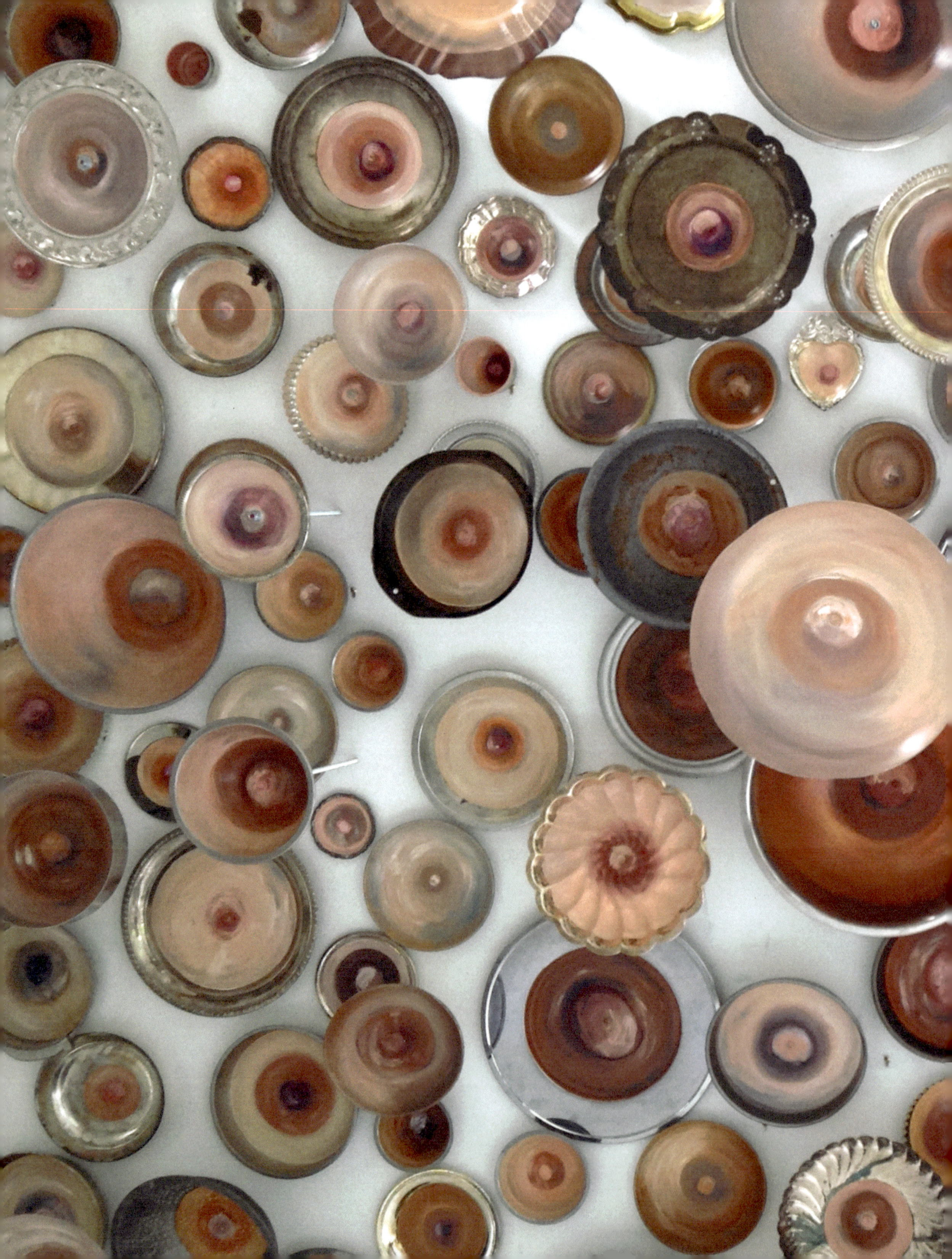

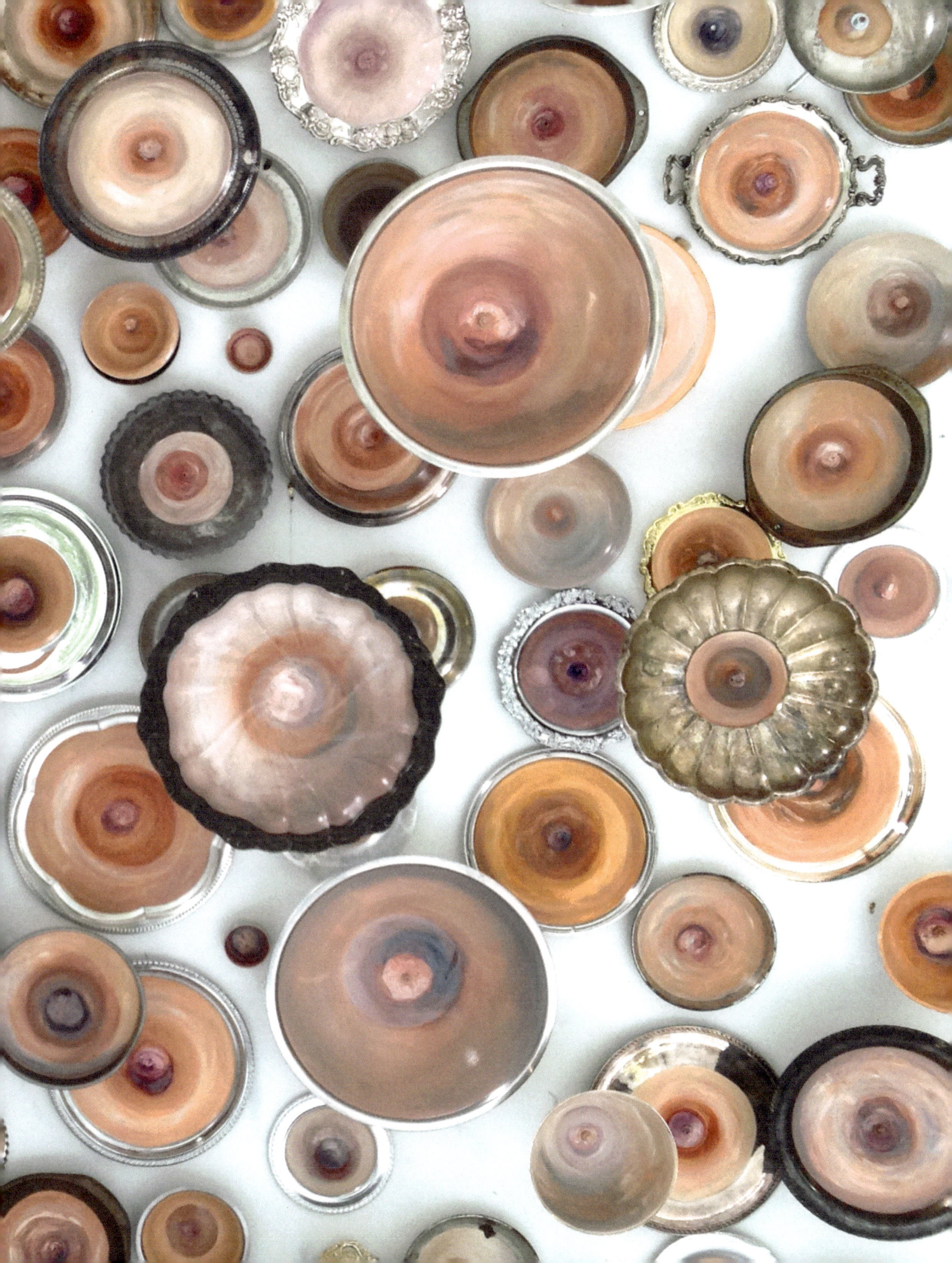

Previous pages
Tit Wall
2014–2015, 144" x 120"
Installation of metal bowls and oil paint

I painted on any round bowl, cake pan or serving dish I could find for about six months. There was tremendous variety in the bowls — silver, sterling, brass, copper, tin, and aluminum. These are vessels that women touch. Their variety and their wear all symbolize the different women affected by cancer.

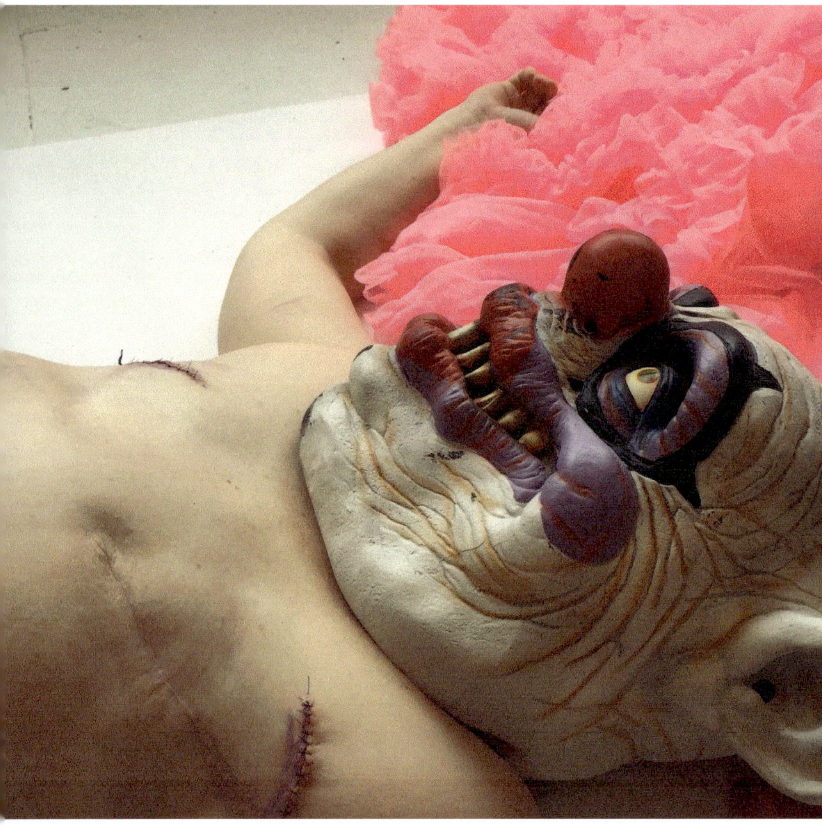

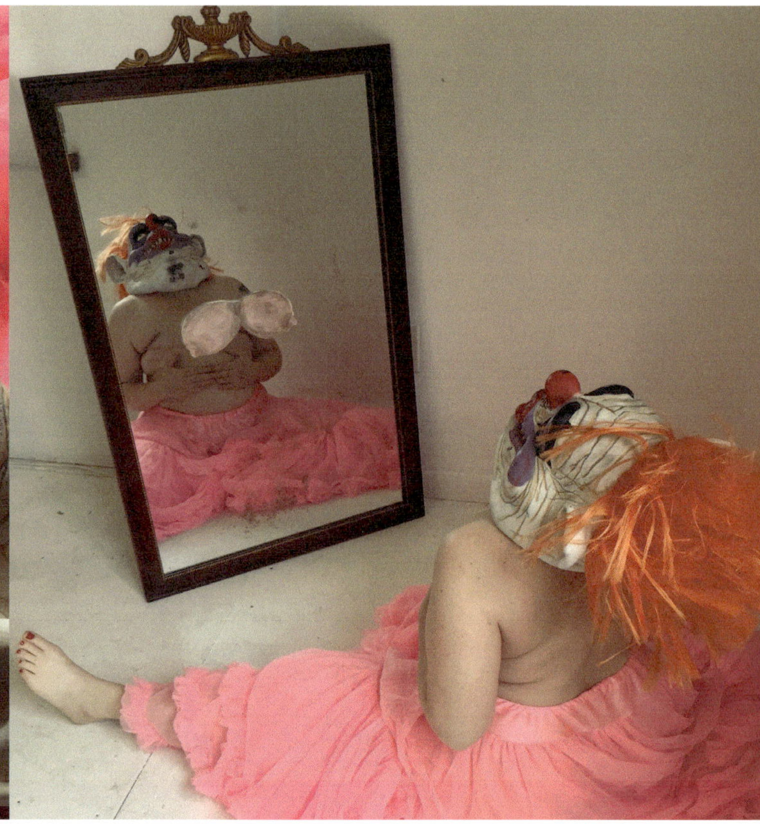

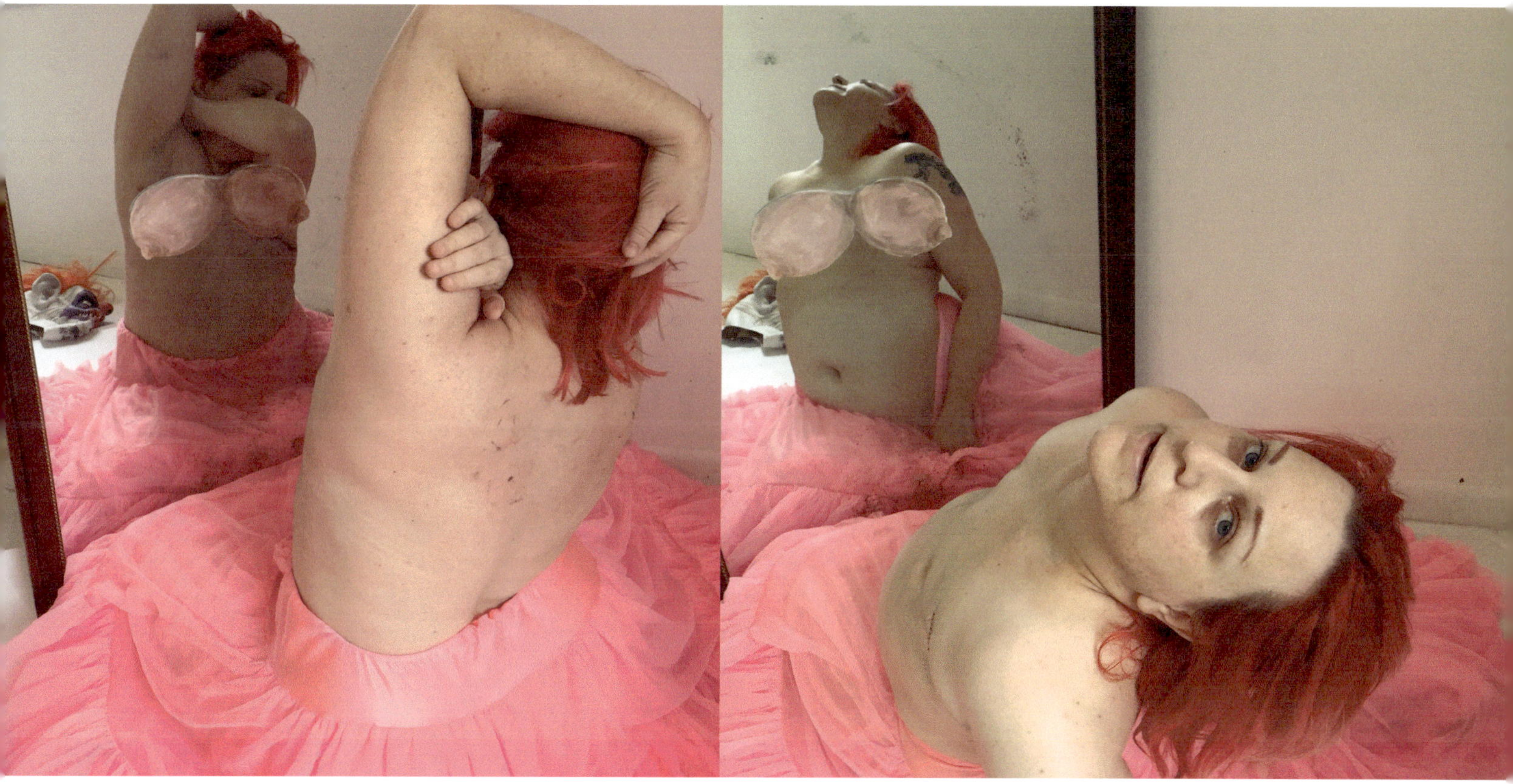

Vanity
2015
Performance, painted mirrors

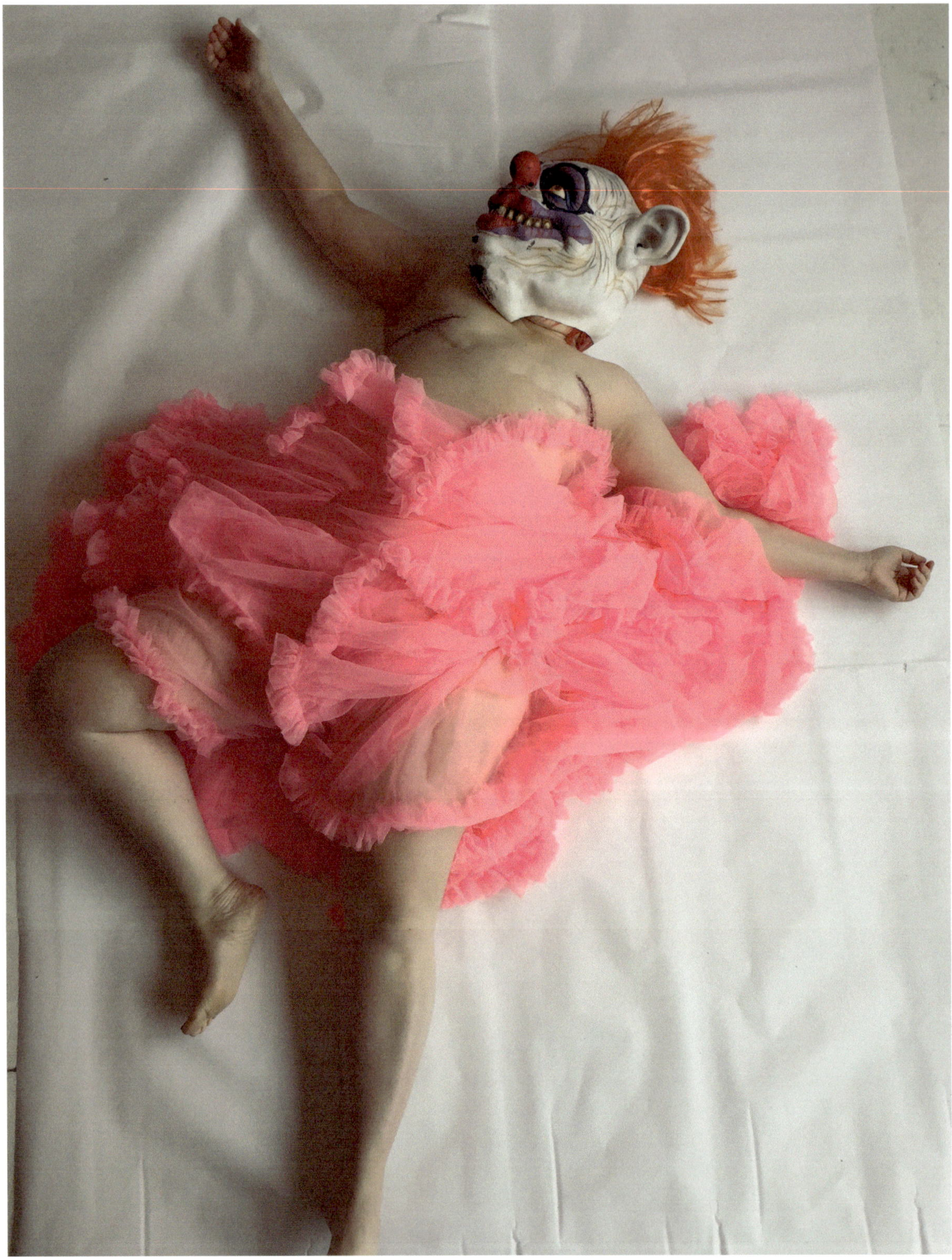

Revision
2015

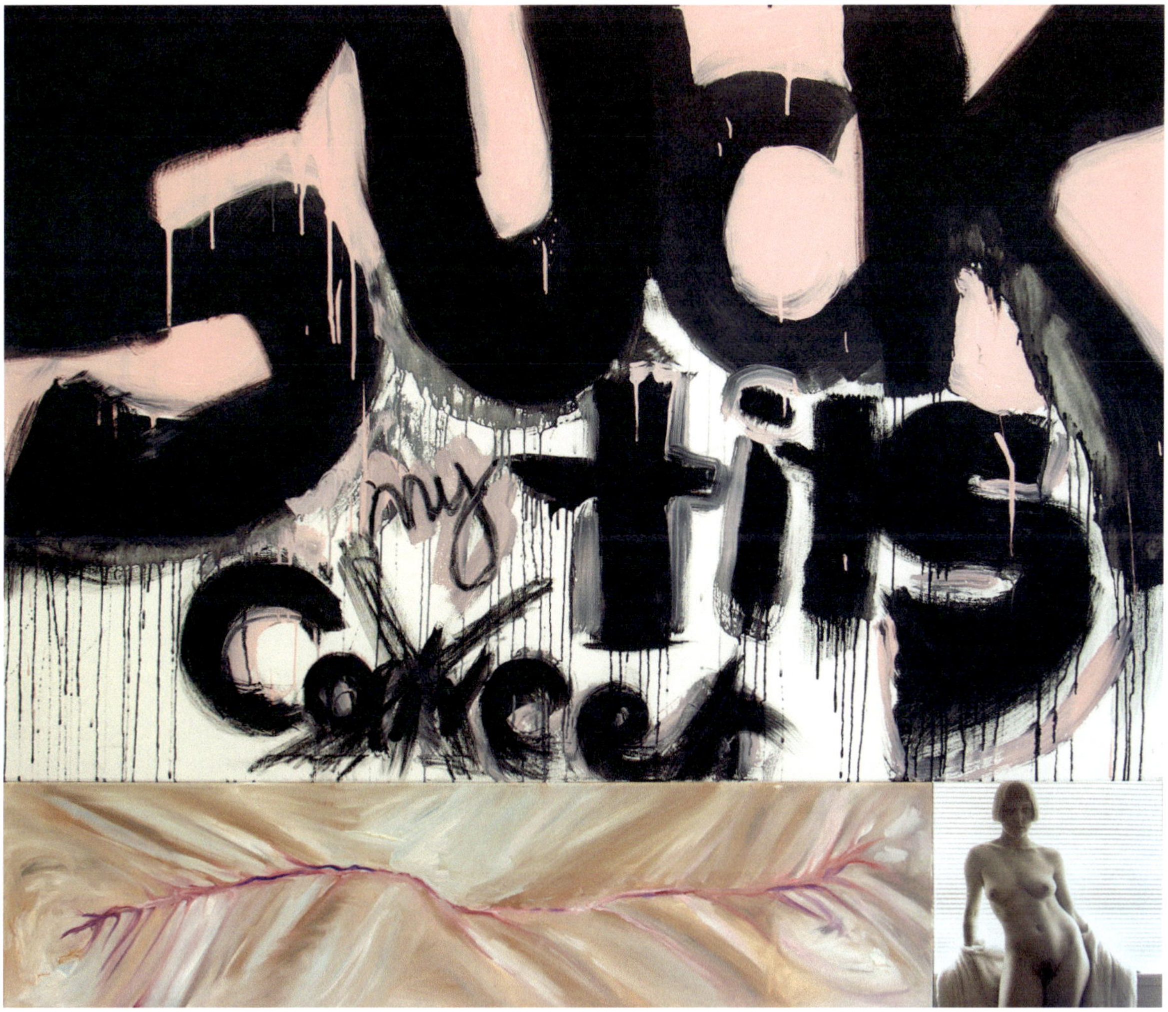

Suck My Tits
2015, 60" x 52"
Oil on canvas, injet on canvas

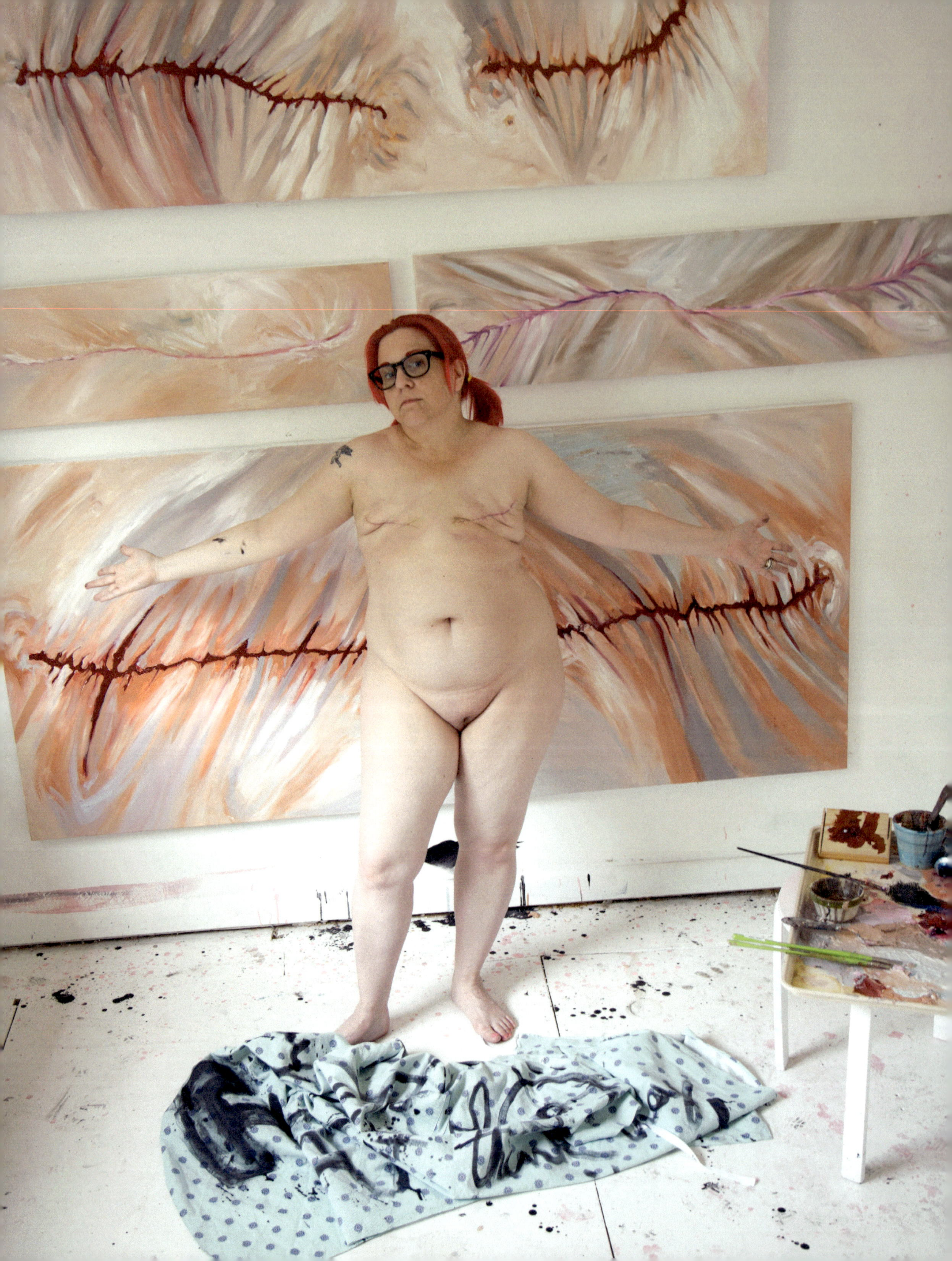

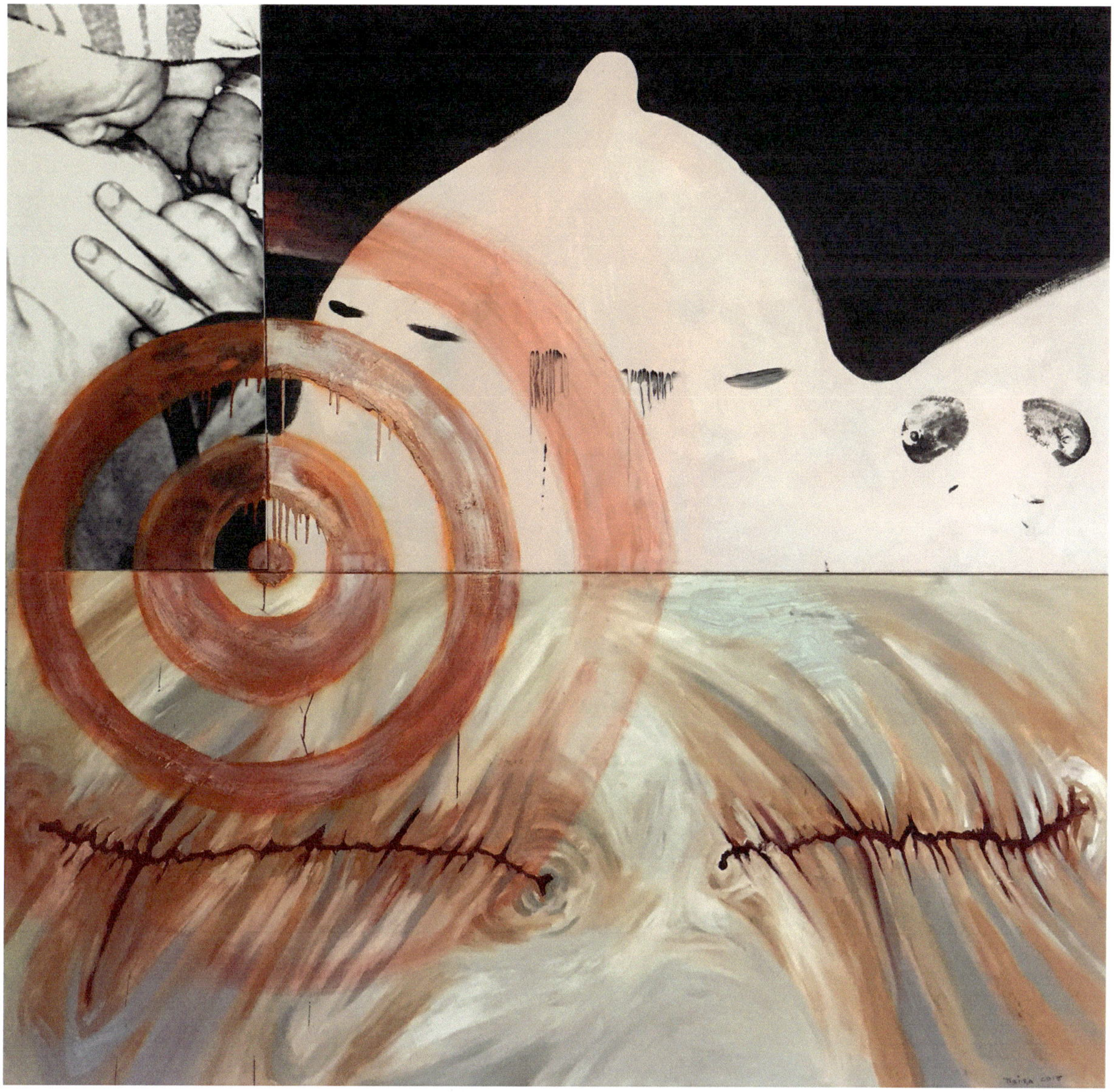

Random Target
2015, 78" x 76"
Oil on canvas, inkjet on canvas

(opposite)
Photo: Jan Johnson

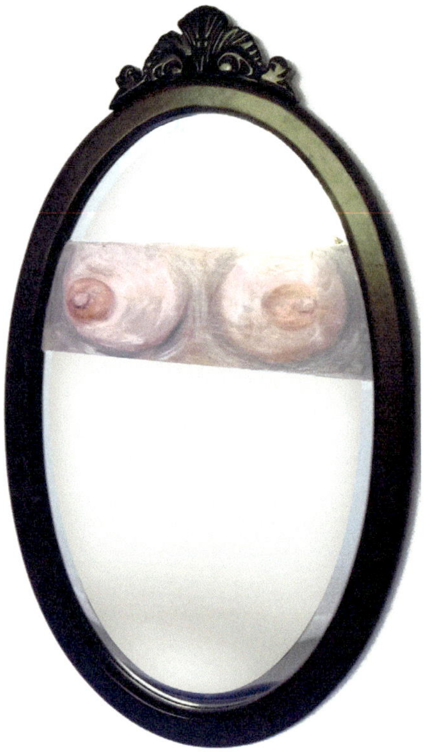

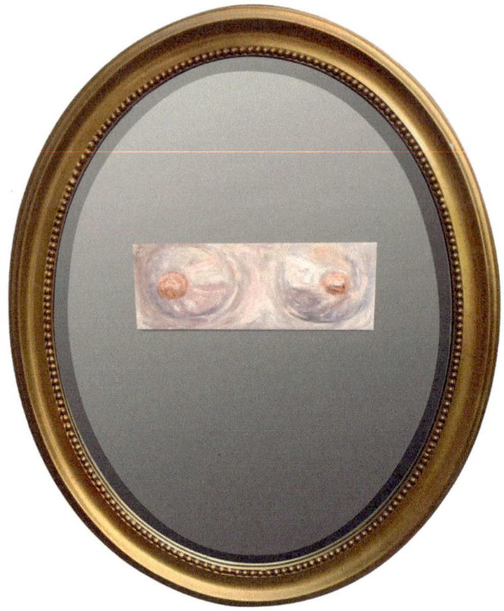

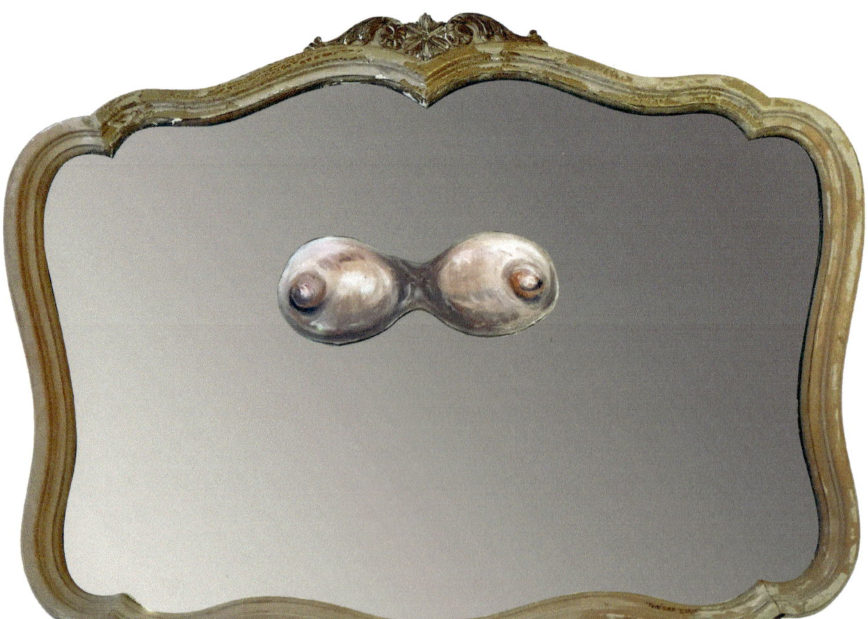

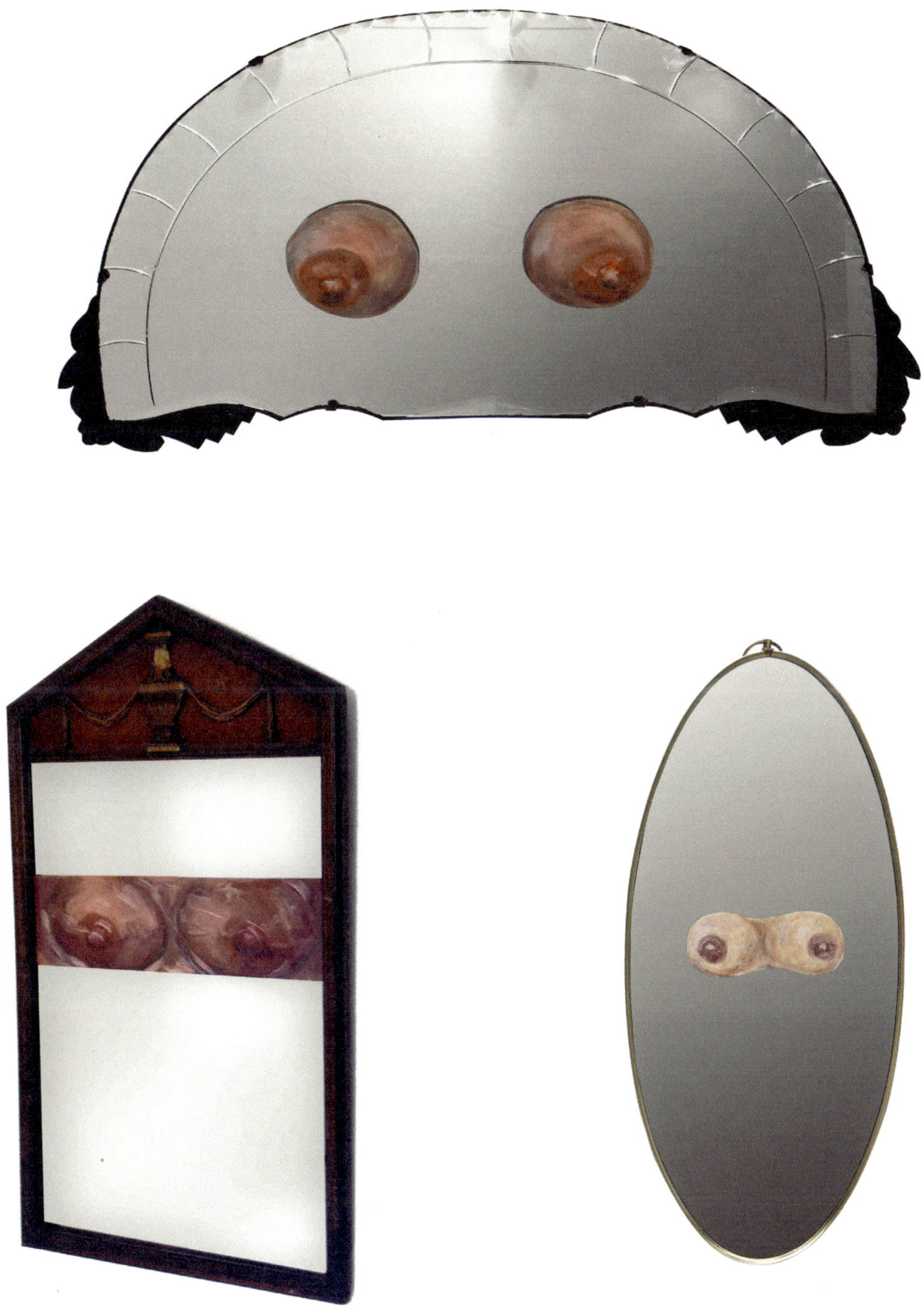

Vanity
2015, sizes vary
Oil on mirrors

February 11, 2014

Dear Thedra,

Thank you for sending your evolving portfolio on your breast cancer to us. First, I love your images. They so clearly (and yes, beautifully) convey your relationship with this disease directed process you are living through. You speak for MANY women who have ridden this roller coaster – but, you are fortunate to have this gift of expression. I know that many other women would find this young series very meaningful and valuable in their own journeys. Even perhaps more importantly is what you can convey to those "surrounding " the woman with the new diagnosis of breast cancer – at least to me you are very clear in the staccato delivery, then processing, of new information and the decisions that must be made that follows that new data. Very beautifully articulated.

Thank you for doing this. I realize it is part of your own "therapy" but it also helps me as a physician and surgeon. I certainly never doubted you were a serious artist (checked your website long ago J) . I look forward to seeing this body of work continue to grow – with downs and ups – to its positive end.

Best wishes – see you next week.

Barbara

Barbara Lee Bass MD, FACS
Chair, Department of Surgery
John F. and Carolyn Bookout Distinguished Endowed Chair
Houston Methodist Hospital
Executive Director
MITIE: The Methodist Institute for Technology, Innovation and Education
Professor of Surgery
Weill Cornell Medical College of Cornell University

6550 Fannin St., Ste. 1661
Houston, TX 77030
713.441.5133
bbass@houstonmethodist.org
www.methodisthealth.com
www.mitietexas.com

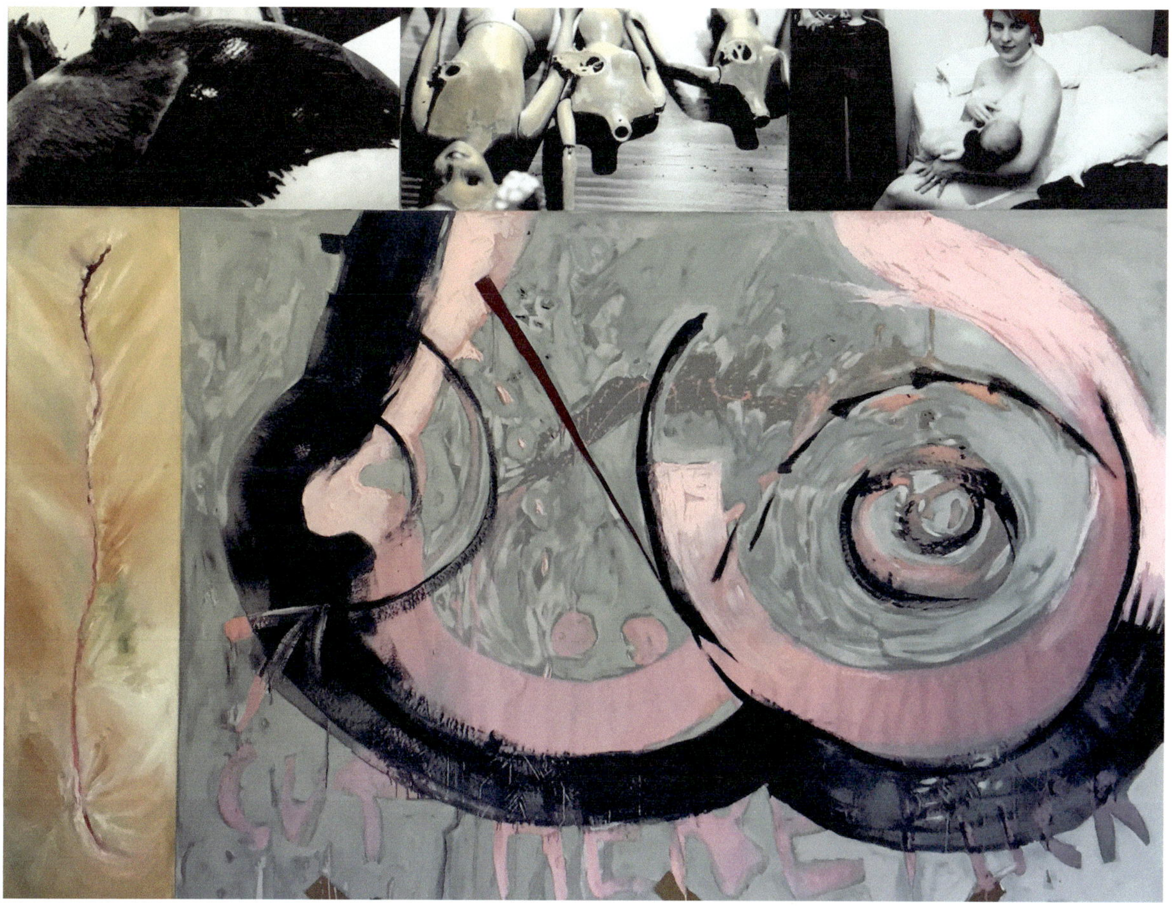

Cut Here 2
2015, 80" x 62"
Oil on canvas, inkjet on canvas

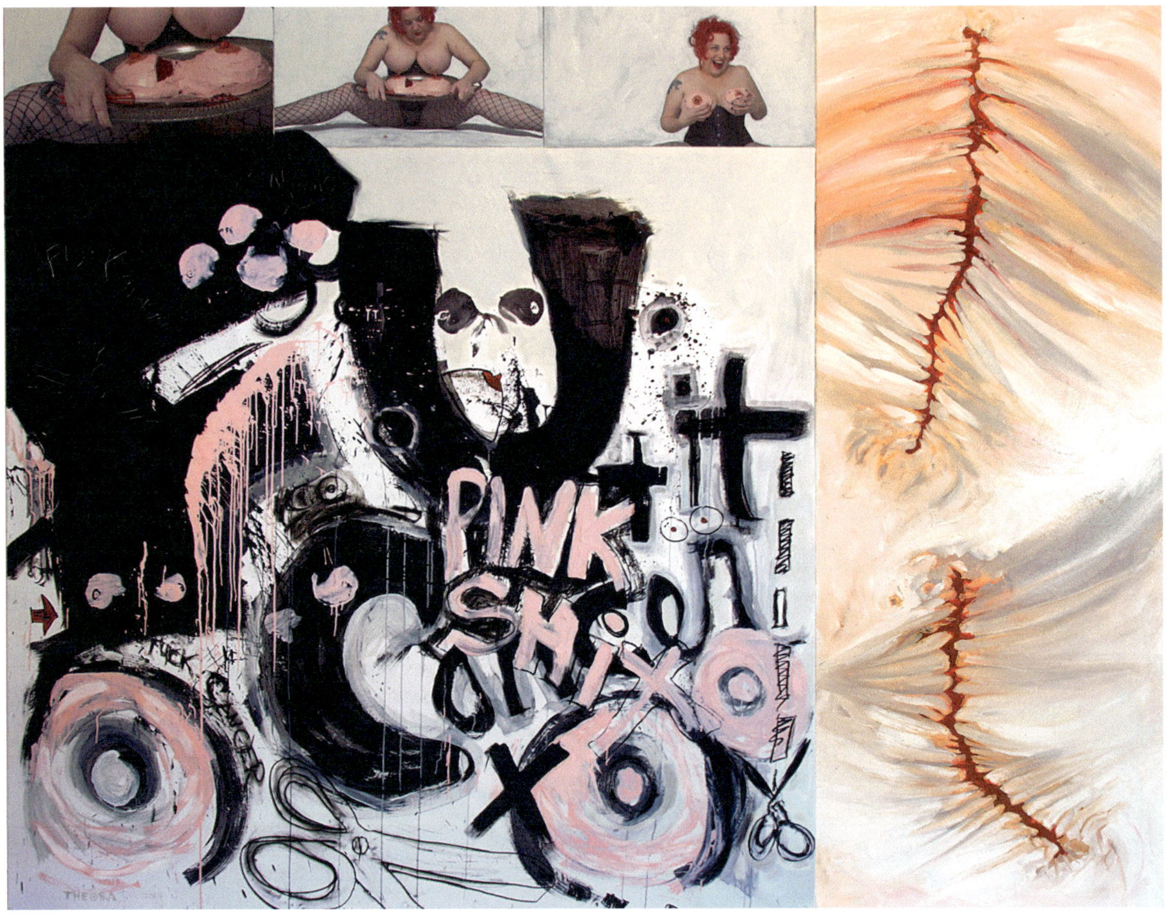

FU Pink Shit
2015, 80" x 64"
Oil on canvas, inkjet on canvas

Whether or not to have breast reconstruction is your decision.

Following a mastectomy, all women should be provided the opportunity to decide for themselves whether or not to have breast reconstruction.

Reasons to rebuild

For any number of reasons, you and/or your loved ones may strongly prefer your appearance with breasts.

You may not feel "whole" without having breasts

If you are clothed, other people will not be able to tell that you had a mastectomy.

Women's fashions will generally fit better.

Reasons not to rebuild

Reconstruction usually requires many surgical procedures, each involving pain, recovery time, and expense.

Surgery cannot restore the sensation of your original breasts and in many cases you will not have a nipple.

Some women find implants uncomfortable or painful. They also may need to be replaced later on.

Inappropriately strong pressure to rebuild (or not to rebuild) can sometimes come from society at-large, friends, family, even from the medical team. Each woman should think carefully about whether breast reconstruction is right for her.

www.facebook.com/groups/FlatANDFabulous

Thank you!

Houston Methodist Hospital (my transplant coordinator Jennifer Hamilton, cancer surgeon Dr. Barbara Bass and Mashonda Garner, oncologist Dr. Angel Rodriguez and his staff, and the Methodist Foundation for their generosity.) The Holly Rose Ribbon Foundation for cleaning up my "dog ears" to make me nice and flat. Thank you for listening to what I really wanted and respecting me as a person (Cindi and Dr. Franklin Rose, Cassie, Ginger, Pam, Stacey, Autumn, and Stephanie.) Gottlieb Foundation NYC, The Rose Mobile Mammograms (Dorothy Gibbons, Jeanne Gillen, and Amy Rigsby), Proud Pony International (Jarrod Gullett and Travis Johns) for video production, T&T Shirts (Ashley), Houston Giclee Printing (David Miller), The Little Piñata Shop, What's Up Cupcake (Laurel Keith), Sargent Joe Henning, Richardean Bartee at Grungecake, G Gallery (Wayne & Beverly Gilbert and Bradford Moody), Poppi Massey for sponsoring the inflatable boob, Interactive Exhibits LLC (Myles Rose), Mark and Carrie Pillsbury for PR, Kimberly DeLape for helping with sponsorships, Mary Magsamen & Stephan Hillerbrand, Catherine Colangelo, Maureen McNamara, Bill Arning, Mark McCray, Rick Herron, Patrick Renner, Everett Taasevigen, Regina Vigil, Mitch Pengra, Kelly Gale Amen, Alicia Kahn, Kayci Wheatley for help with merch and decades of friendship, Boston Bostian, Laura Conely, Michael Mueller, Michael Stewart, Sherry & Robert Hughes, Dania Dandashli, The Flat and Fabulous Group on Facebook (founded by Barbie Ritzo and Sarah Bartosiewicz-Hamilton) Christine Brown, Shelly Marie Williams-Griffith, Bettina Desrochers, Debb Summers, Shelly Marie, Sarah Brandon, Pennie Coss Yugmang, Melanie Testa, Cambria Dodd Russell, Heidi Brubaker Cooper, Zury Baca, the Queer Cancer group (Emily Jensen, Uta Melle, Loony Loo, Juanita Noons Shaw), and all of my flat and fabulous sisters for keeping me sane. Finally, Carol Cullar, Nan Jenkins & Timmi Kuykendall, Loden & Heather, Sage, and Stephen Cullar-Ledford.

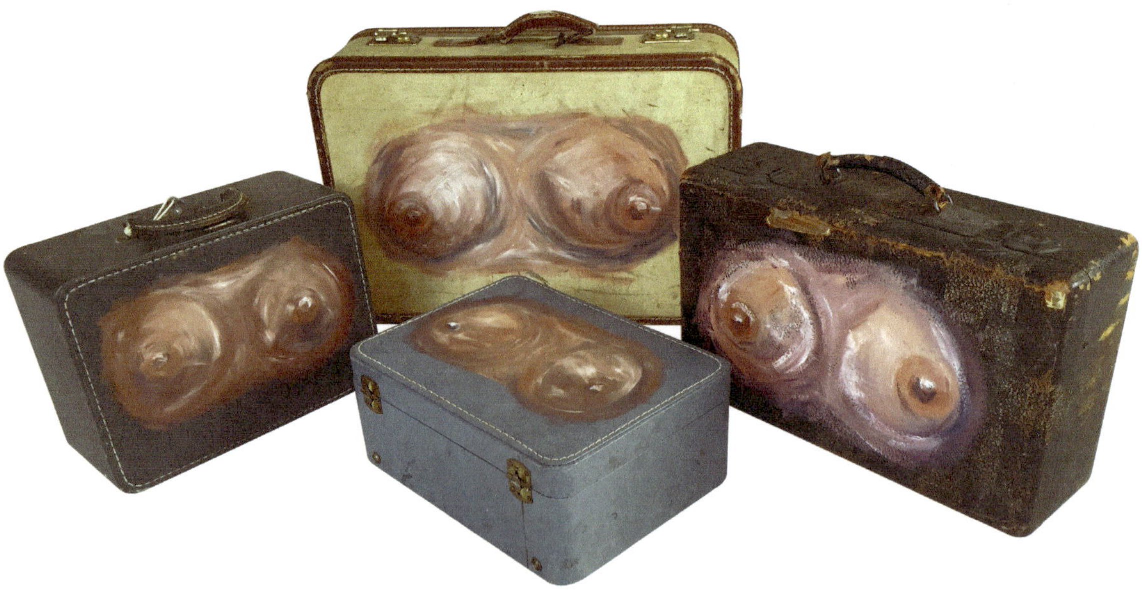

Pack Up Your Troubles
2015, dimensions vary
Oil on found suitcases

Opposite:
Photo: Everett Taasevigen

Made in the USA
Monee, IL
12 September 2026

62979089R00043